HERBS
An Herbal Reference Guide

Henry Hernandez

Copyright © 2018 Henry Hernandez

All rights reserved.

ISBN: 172283868X
ISBN-13: 978-1722838683

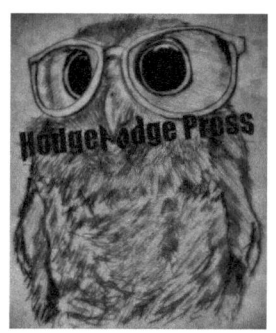

I would like to dedicate this book to my great-grandfather, who passed his knowledge and healing abilities on to me so I could continue his work, passing his knowledge of healing herbs to others.

To my metaphysical instructor, Ricardo, for opening up my heart to the beautiful world of spiritualism and opening up my mind to greater understanding of my great-grandfather's knowledge to help and heal others.

To all the men and women who have served this country and paid the ultimate price defending it.

And last by not least, to my beautiful friend, Shannon, who made this book possible so I could pass on my ancestral knowledge.

DISCLAIMER

Always consult your physician before taking any herbal remedies. Never stop taking your prescribed medications without consulting with your physician first.

TABLE OF CONTENTS

1	Herbal Terminology	Page 1
2	Medicinal Herb Preparations	Page 4
3	Adaptogen	Page 10
4	Alterative	Page 18
5	Digestive	Page 26
6	Nervines	Page 34
7	Respiratory	Page 43
8	Reproductive	Page 50
9	General Index	Page 66
10	References	Page 68

Herbal Terminology

Adaptogen - An herb that strengthens or rejuvenates the system.

Alterative - Blood purifying herbs. They aid in riding the blood of metabolic waste products and in absorb nutrients. They are high in minerals and some vitamins.

Alkaloid - Group of organic, alkaline compounds that contain nitrogen.

Amphoteric - An herb that works on both aspects of a health problem, ex. high or low blood pressure.

Analgesic - A pain relieving herb, both internal and externally. They are less potent than prescribed anesthetics or narcotics.

Antibiotic - Herbs that are used to kill bacterial germs.

Anthelmintic - An herb that destroys or rids the body of intestinal worms.

Antipyretic - An herb that helps to reduce fever.

Antiseptic - An herb that helps to prevent the growth of bacteria.

Antispasmodic - An herb that helps to relieve spasms or cramps.

Aperient - A laxative

Aperitif - An agent that stimulates appetite.

Astringent - An herb that contracts tissue. It is used to control bleeding or decrease secretions.

Carminative - An herb that relaxes the stomach and stimulates peristalsis. It also aids in relieving gas.

Catarrh - An inflammation of the mucous membrane.

Cathartic - Relieves constipation

Cholagogue - An herb that helps secrete bile.

Demulcent - An oily or gelatinous substance that soothes inflamed or irritated tissue.

Diaphoretic - An herb that induces sweating by stimulating the kidneys when taken hot. When it is taken cold, it acts as a diuretic.

Emetic - Induces vomiting

Emmenagogue - An herb that promotes menstrual flow.

Emollient - An herb that is applied externally to soften and sooth the skin.

Expectorant - An herb that expels excess mucous from the respiratory tract.

Galactagogue/Lactagogue - An herb that increases secretion of milk.

Hemostatic - An agent that stops internal bleeding.

Hepatics - An herb that helps tone, strengthen, and increase the flow of bile.

Lithotripics - An herb that dissolves and eliminates urinary and biliary stones.

Maceration - A process of softening the tissues by soaking in liquid.

Menstruum - A substance that dissolves a solid or holds it in suspension.

Mucilage - A gelatinous substance that soothes inflammation. The substance contains proteins and polysaccharides.

Nervine - An herb that calms tension, nervousness, or excitement.

Poultice - A moist combination of herbs, or single herb, applied to the skin to provide healing moisture and heat.

Salve - An herbal preparation applied to the skin after being mixed in oil and thickened with beeswax.

Tincture - An herbal solution prepared by steeping or soaking plant material in Vodka, apple cider vinegar, or vegetable glycerin.

Vulnerary - An herb that heals the body by promoting cell growth and repair. It is mainly used when dealing with wounds.

Medicinal Herb Preparations

Harvesting, Drying, and Storing Medicinal Herbs

Harvesting Herbs

    a) The best time to harvest herbs is at 10am after the dew has dried off the plant. The evening time is also optimal. Avoid any harvesting during the midday heat.
    b) It's ideal to snip the aerial stems between the nodes.
    c) Harvesting in the fall is ideal.

Drying Herbs

    a) For herbs with long stems, tie the stems together and hang them upside down in a well-ventilated room.
    b) You can place leaved herbs between folded paper towels to dry them.
    c) The drying process is done when you can crumble the herb between your fingers. Do not over dry your herbs because they will lose their potency.

Storing Herbs

    a) Once the drying process of your herbs is complete, pull the herbs off the stem or crumble them.
    b) Store your herbs in an airtight glass container.
    c) Keep your herbs in a dark pantry or cabinet.
    d) Label all your jars with the herb's name and date.
    e) Properly stored herbs can stay fresh for 1 to 2 years.

Preparing Medicinal Teas

The two different types of medicinal teas are infusion and decoction. An infusion is made from the soft parts of the herb (leaves and flowers). A decoction is made from the hard parts of the herb (roots, stems, and berries). Even though medicinal teas are brewed with hot water, you can drink them hot, at room temperature, or cold, and still receive their medicinal properties. Always use a stainless steel, glass, or ceramic kettle or pot when preparing your teas. Don't use copper or aluminum as it will negatively affect the quality of the herb.

Medicinal Infusion

   a) Bring water to a boil in your kettle.
   b) Measure your herb: fresh herb (2 tablespoons) or dried herb (1 tablespoons) per cup of water.
   c) Pour the necessary cups of water over the measured herbs, cover the teapot or steeping pot, and let the herbs infuse for 15 minutes.
   d) Strain and drink.
   e) Consume the tea in a mug 3 times per day

Medicinal Decoction

   a) Add a desired amount of cold water to a pot.
   b) Place cut roots, stems, or berries (2 to 3 tablespoons per quart of water) in a pot, and bring to a boil.
   c) Once the water is boiling, cover, and reduce the heat and simmer for 20 minutes.
   d) Strain and drink.
   e) Consume the tea in a mug 3 times per day

Herbal Tincture

An herbal tincture is an herbal preparation that is taken internally for a variety of medical concerns. Tinctures are primarily made with a vodka menstruum. Menstruum is a liquid medium that draws out the medicinal properties of the herb and holds the herbs in suspension. You can also use apple cider vinegar or vegetable glycerin as your menstruum.

a) Place fresh, wilted, chopped, or dried herbs into a glass jar with a tight-fitting lid.
b) Add the menstruum of your choice, completely covering the herbs but leaving an inch to an inch-and-a-half of free space at the top of the jar.
c) If you are using vegetable glycerin as your menstruum, mix with equal parts of distilled water. If using vinegar, warm the vinegar first before pouring it over the herb.
d) Store the jar in a warm, dark place and let it steep/macerate for 6 to 8 weeks.
e) Shake the jar daily.
f) After the steeping period is up, strain the herb from the menstruum and store the tincture in dark bottles in a cool, shaded area.
g) Label the bottle with name and date.

Tinctures can be administered under the tongue or diluted in tea, water, or juice. Tinctures can also be used externally as a liniment or rub.

An alcohol-based tincture can keep for many years. A glycerin tincture will keep for 2 to 3 years, and a vinegar-based one is good for at least 1 year.

The dose for a tincture is 1 drop for every 5 lbs of body weight.

¼ teaspoon = 1 dropper-full (35 drops) = 1 ml

The typical dose for tinctures is 3 times per day

Salve Making

Salves are used externally for various skin problems, such as eczema, psoriasis, rashes, burns, cuts, wounds, insect bites, and more.

1) Place fresh, wilted or dried herbs into a glass jar. Add extra virgin olive oil (EVOO), allowing for two inches of oil to cover the herbs. This will make an infused oil.
2) Set the jar on a window sill in indirect sunlight for two weeks.
3) Strain herbs from the oil with a stainless-steel strainer.
4) Pour the oil into a glass measuring cup.
5) Place the strained, measured oil into a double boiler on a low heat.
6) Add chopped or grated beeswax to the oil. The measurement is one part beeswax to four parts oil. To check the consistency of the oil, place one teaspoon of oil in the refrigerator for 3 minutes. Take it out and check the salve. If it is too soft, add more beeswax; if it is too hard, add more oil.
7) When you reach the desired consistency, you can add Vitamin E and/or any essential oils you may choose (optional).
8) Pour into small containers with tight-fitting lids.
9) Label jars with product name and date.
10) Store salve in a cool, dry place. Exposing the salve to extreme heat will weaken it and cause it to spoil quickly.

ADAPTOGEN

Ashwaganda   **Adaptogen & Reproductive**

Winter Cherry, Indian Ginseng

Parts Used: Root (Capsules, Powder)

Native to India

Helps with stress, anxiety, depression, panic attacks, insomnia, behavioral problems, poor memory, concentration, ADHD, loss of energy and muscular strength, arthritis and insomnia due to advanced age; slows aging process; boosts male virility hindered by age and decreased testosterone levels; anti-inflammatory for joint problems; enhances immunity; promotes sleep.

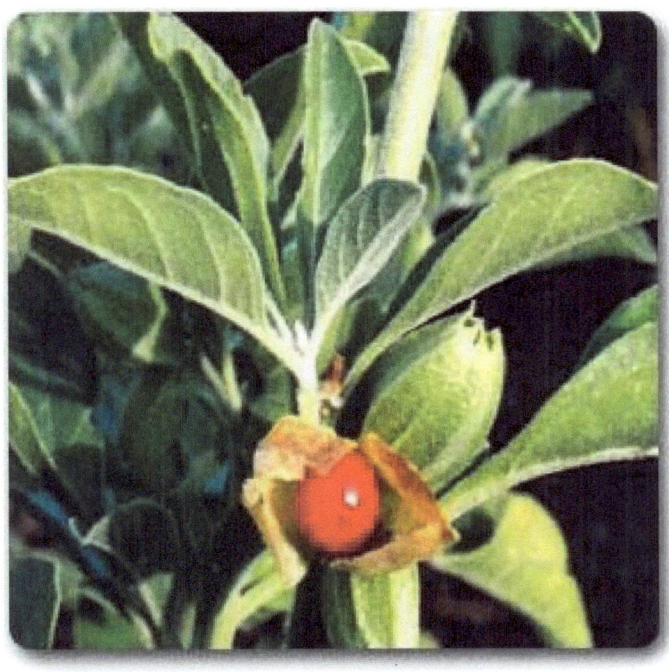

Astragalus

Astragalus Root, Yellow Leader

Astragalus membranaceus

Parts Used: Root (Decoction, Tincture, Capsules)

Native to Northeast China

Used for cold, flu, minor infections, dry cough, asthma, angina, atherosclerosis, bladder infection; restores T-cell function in cancer patients and prevents growth in cancerous cells; regulates diabetes; stimulates the activity of T-helper cells depleted by AIDS, infertility, lupus, rheumatoid arthritis, Myasthenia Gravis.

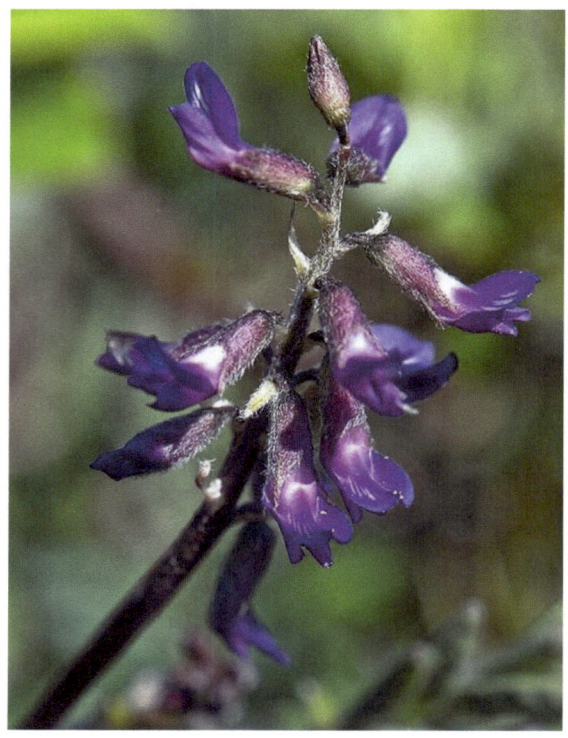

Cleavers

Clivers, Goose Grass, Cathch Weed, Sweet Woodruff

Galium aparine

Parts Used: Aerial Parts (Infusion, Tincture)

Native to Europe

Enhances lymph circulation; reduces inflammation and heat to an inflamed area; helps with arthritis and gout; promotes immune function; diuretic; eases UTIs and irritable bladder; lowers blood pressure; improves digestion; stimulates bile flow.

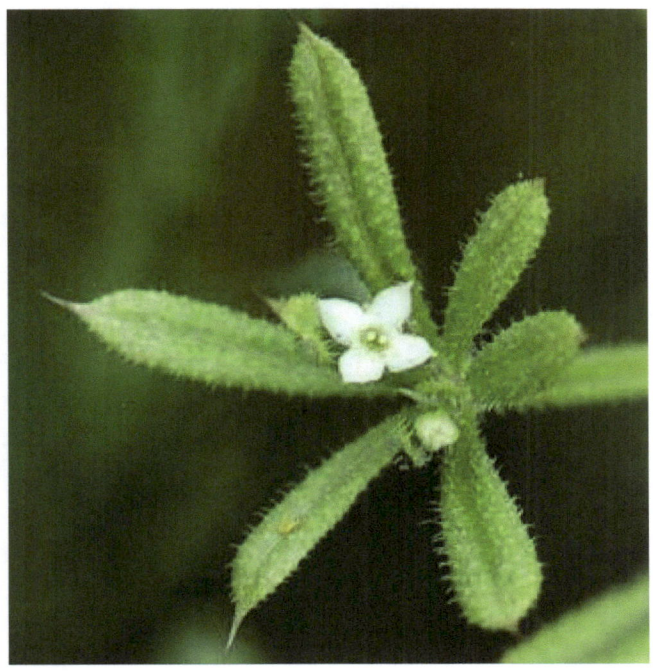

Eleuthero

Siberian Ginseng, Russian Ginseng, Touch-me-not

Eleutherococcus senticosus

Parts Used: Root (Tincture, Capsules)

Native to Northern Asia

Improves digestion and absorption of nutrients; increases strength; relieves lethargy; increases stamina; helps decrease stress levels, jet lag; increases mental stamina in those with ADHD and failing memory; relieves adrenal fatigue; disposes of lactic acid; enhances immune system against infection and viruses.

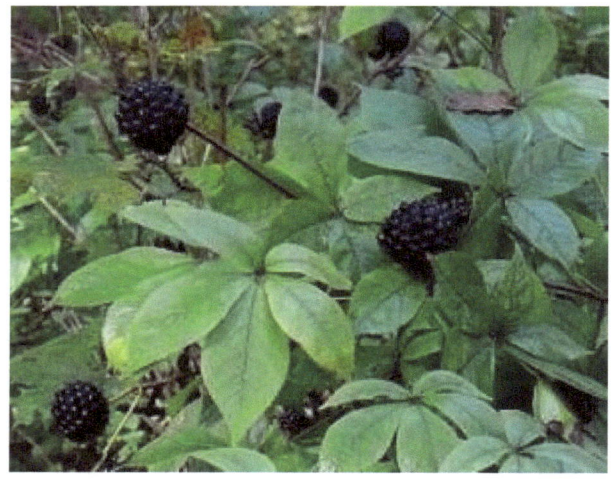

He Shou Wu

Fo-Ti, Ho Shou Wu

Polygonum multiflorum

Parts Used: Root (Capsules)

Native to China

Supports liver and kidney detox; treats infertility, premature aging, weakness, vaginal discharge; high in Zinc; mild sedative qualities to calm nervous system; anti-inflammatory; supports blood building and blood-cell health with Iron; strengthens kidneys, adrenals, mental clarity; improves low back and knee pain associated with kidney deficiency; helps strengthen muscles and tendons; improves sleep; reduces high cholesterol and blood pressure.

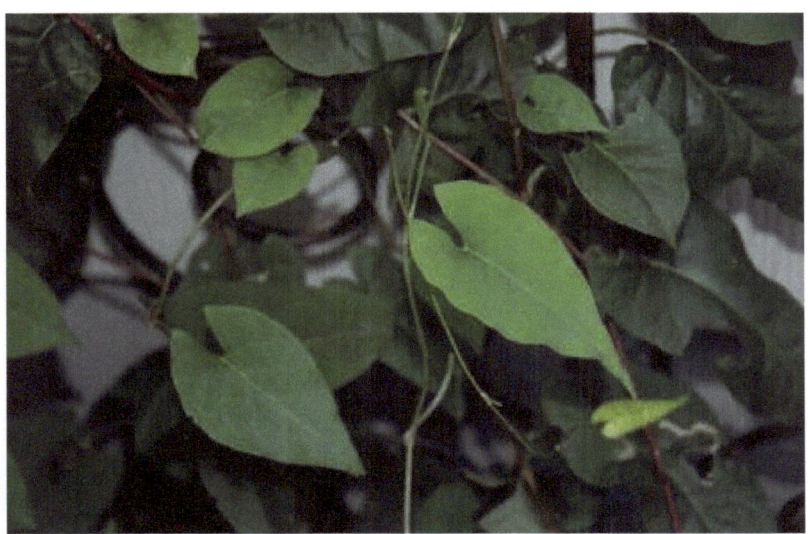

Holy Basil

Tulsi, Tulasi, Indian Basil

Ocimum sanctum

Parts Used: Whole Plant (Infusion, Tincture, Powder)

Native to India

Antispasmodic; improves digestive absorption; used for anorexia, nausea, constipation, vomiting, abdominal pain, ulcers and worms; increases production of stomach mucous, mental clarity; reduces anxiety, mild depression, insomnia, stress-related problems such as headaches and irritable bowel syndrome; decongestant; expectorant; helps with asthma, rhinitis, cough, cold, fever, sore throat, flu; protects healthy cells from the toxicity of radiation and chemotherapy, hay fever, dysuria, cystitis; UTIs clear through the diuretic effect; lowers blood sugar, cholesterol and triglyceride levels.

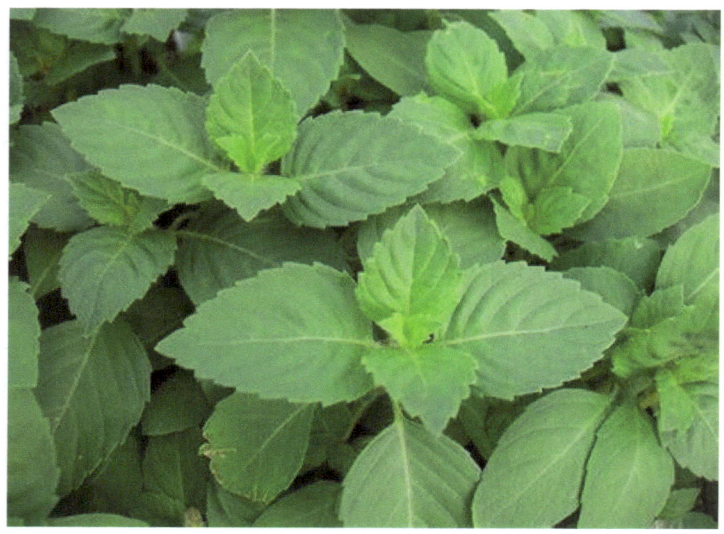

Rhodiola

Golden Root, Rose Root, Arctic Root

Rhodiola rosea

Parts Used: Root, Stem, leaves, Flowers, Seeds (Tincture)

Native to Himalaya

Grows in Northern Hemisphere at high elevations in Asia, Europe, and North America

Helps with altitude sickness, anemia, and cardiovascular disorder; combats the effects of excess adrenaline; stress reliever; increases blood supply to the brain and muscles; increases attention span, memory and mental performance; elevates mood in depression; useful sedative for insomnia in higher doses; eases chronic fatigue syndrome, fibromyalgia; is an energy tonic; increases strength and endurance in athletes and the elderly; stimulates immunity; assists in the prevention of cancer due to its anti-tumor, anti-metastatic, and anti-mutagenic properties; supportive during chemo and radiation therapy; shortens recovery time of suppressed WBCs following chemo.

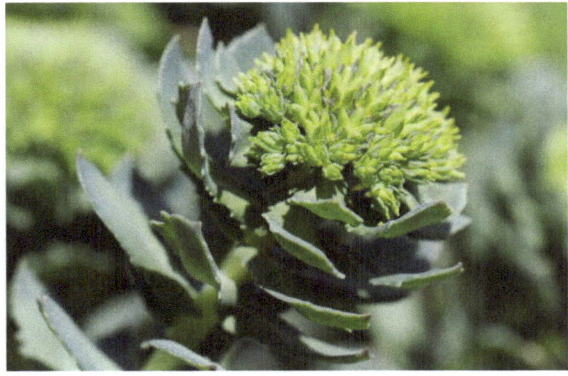

ALTERATIVE

Burdock Root

Gobo, Niv Bang Zi

Arctium lappa

Parts Used: Root, Seed, Leaves (Tincture-Leaves, Root & Seed-Decoction)

Native to Europe and Northern Asia

Enhances digestion and liver function; mild laxative; reduces blood-sugar levels; antibacterial; antiviral; antifungal; reduces fever, acne, boils, eczema, arthritis, fibromyalgia, gout, cystitis, water retention.

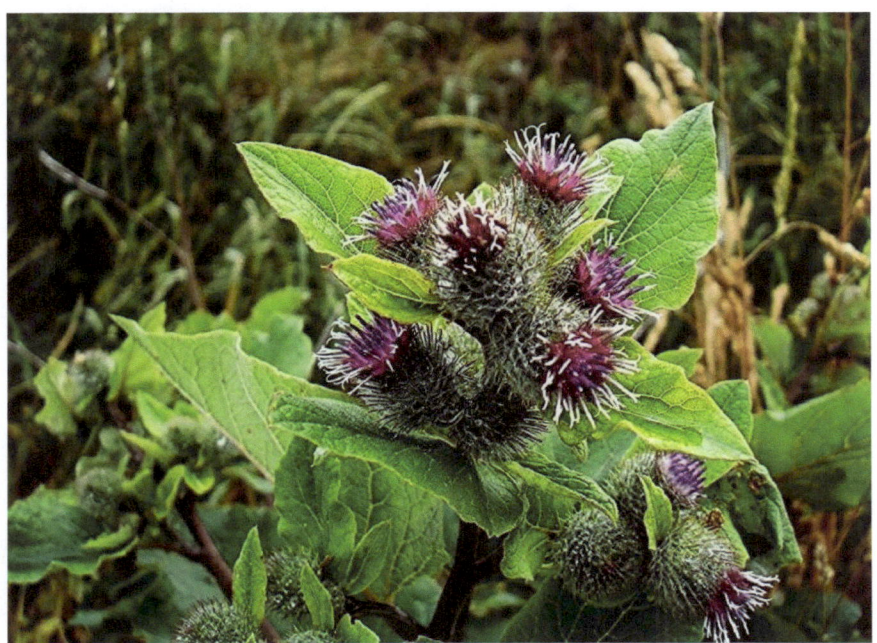

Dandelion

Lion's Tooth

Taraxacum officinale

Parts used: Leaf, Root (Leaf-Infusion and Tincture, Root-Tincture)

Native to Europe, Western Asia and North America

Increases digestive secretions, including bile; stabilizes blood sugar; detoxes liver; diuretic; anti-inflammatory; eases arthritis.

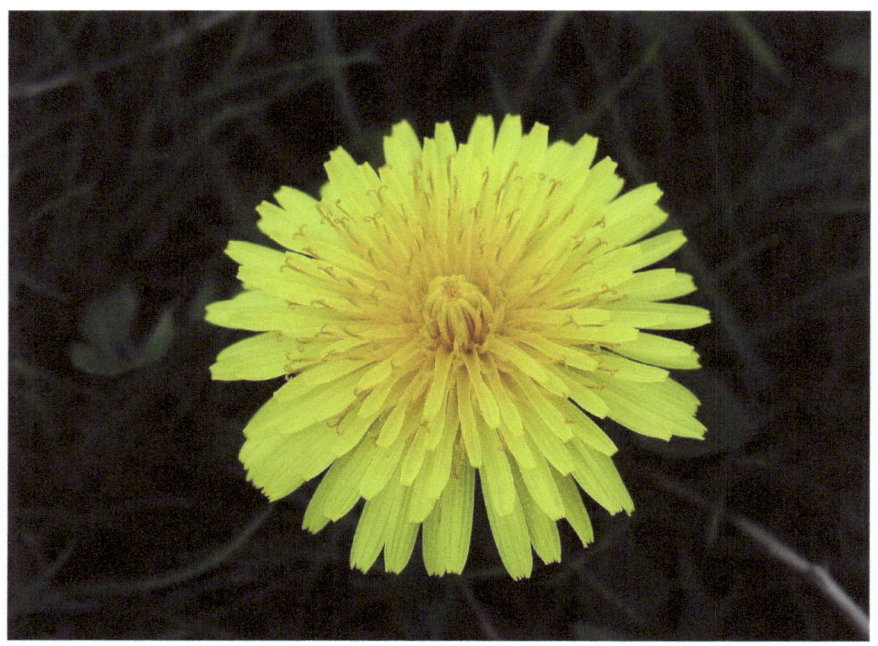

Echinacea

Echinacea Root, Purple Coneflower Root

Echinacea purpurea

Parts Used: Whole Plant (Tincture, Capsules)

Native to North America

Used for colds, flu, viral and bacterial disorders; immune booster; relieves skin disorders such as eczema and acne.

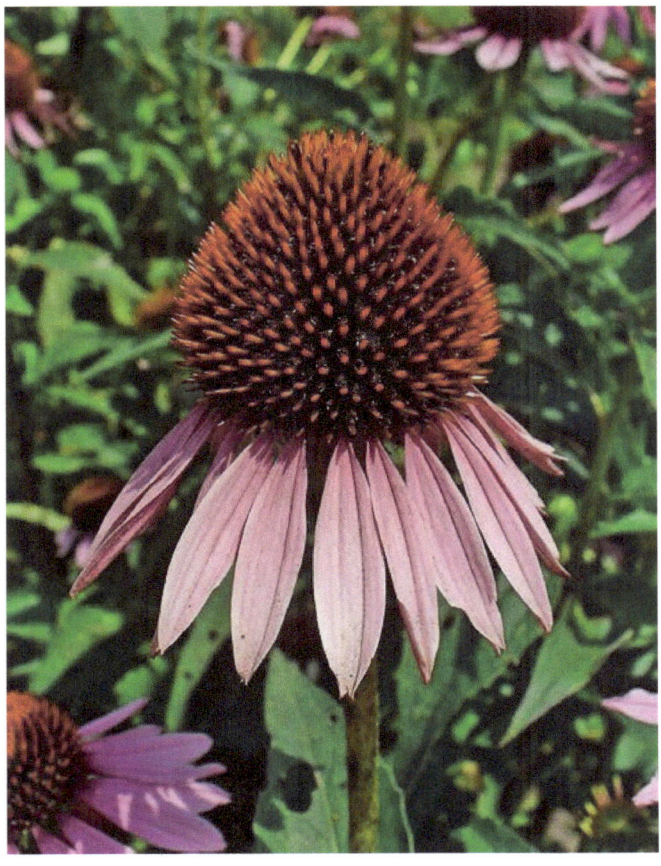

Garlic

Allium satiuum

Parts Used: Clove (Tincture, Infusion)

Antibiotic; antifungal; blood thinner; counters cough and respiratory infections; lowers blood pressure and cholesterol levels; supports beneficial normal flora.

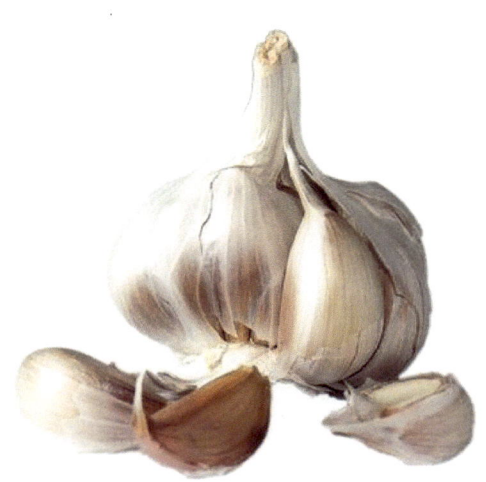

Golden Seal

Yellow Root

Hydrastis canadenis

Parts Used: Root (Tincture, Decoction)

Native to North America

Improves appetite, digestion and absorption; relieves upset stomach, indigestion, gastroenteritis, diarrhea, dysentery; helps with bile flow; detoxes liver, peptic ulcer; re-establishes normal flora; enhances heart function and circulation; raises blood pressure; stimulates production of white blood cells to ward off infection.

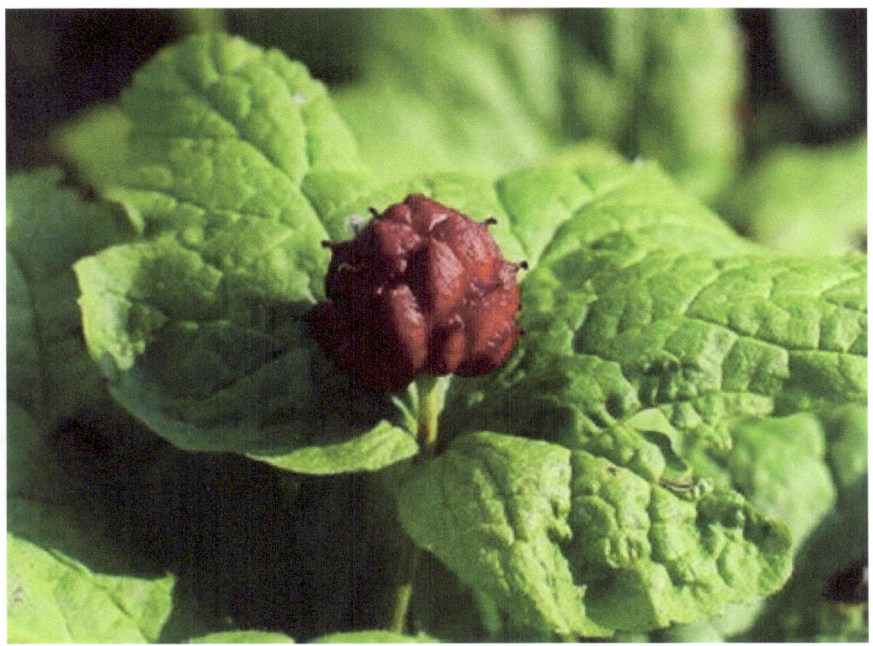

Stinging Nettle   **Alterative, Digestive, Reproductive**

Garden Nettle

Urtica dioica

Parts Used: Leaves, Roots (Infusion-leaf, Tincture-root)

Native to Europe, Asia, North Africa, North America

Protects stomach lining from irritation and infection; relieves diarrhea and flatulence; stimulates liver and kidney function; clears toxins; reduces blood sugar, cough, hay fever, bronchitis, asthma, allergies; stimulates breast milk production; regulates periods and reduces heavy bleeding; rich in Iron; diuretic; prevents incontinence; reduces uric acid for gout; reduces eczema; heals cuts, wounds, hemorrhoids, bites/stings.

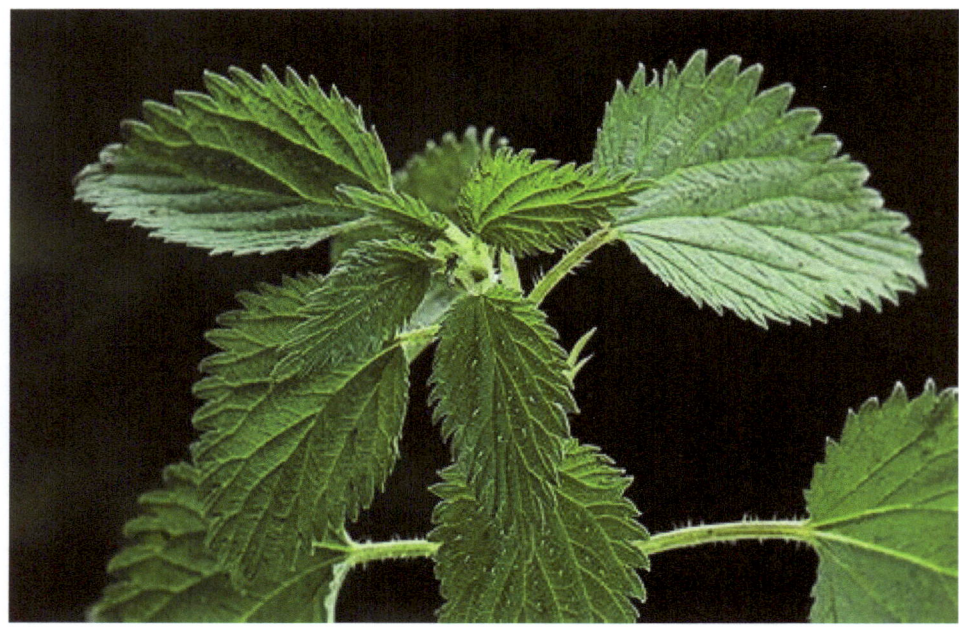

Yellow Dock

Curled Dock, Garden Patience, Sour Dock

Rumex crispus

Parts Used: Root (Tincture, Decoction, Capsule)

Native to Europe and Africa

Laxative; detoxes liver; relieves chronic toxicity and skin disorders such as acne, boils, eczema, and psoriasis.

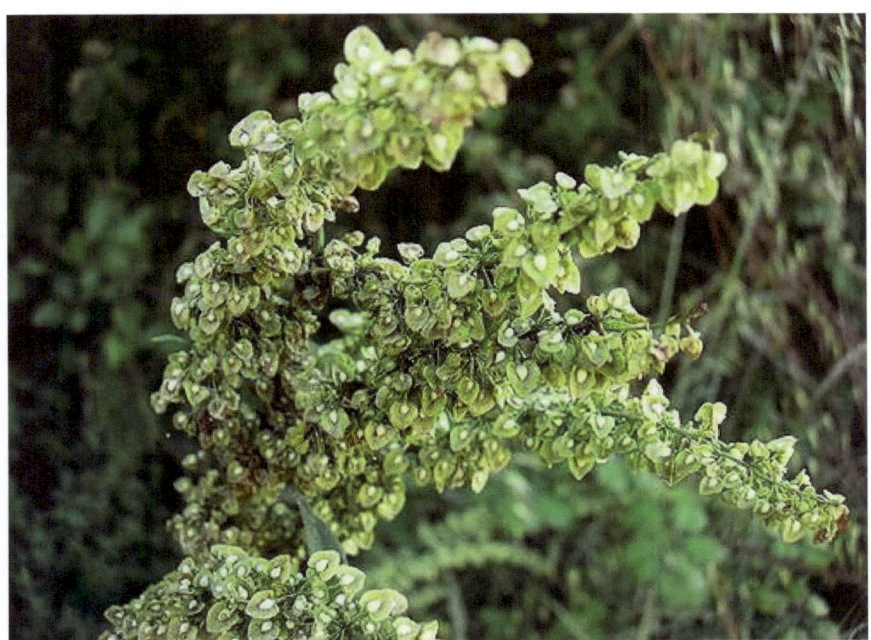

DIGESTIVE

Anise Seed

Aniseed

Pimpinella anisum

Parts Used: Seed (Tincture, Infusion)

Native to Mediterranean Region and Southwest Asia

Reduces flatulence, hiccups, nausea, indigestion, abdominal cramps, asthma, bronchitis, spasmodic coughs; stimulates mother's milk; improves appetite.

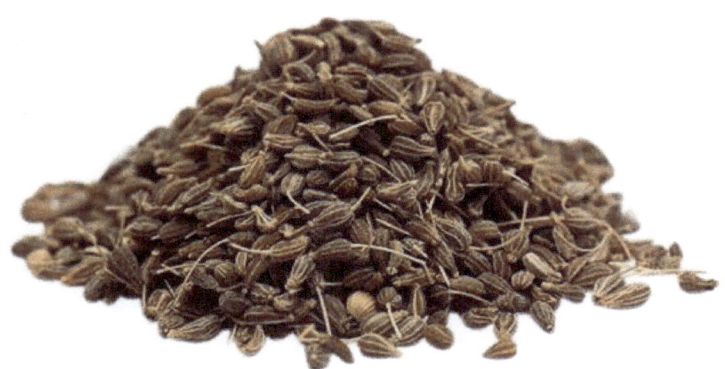

Cascara Sagrada

Buckthorn

Rhamnus purshianus

Parts Used: Bark (Tincture, Decoction)

Native to Western North America, Southern British Columbia, South to Central California, East and Northwest Montana

Aids with indigestion, chronic constipation, inadequate peristalsis. This herb will stimulate the secretions of the whole digestive system including the liver, gall bladder, pancreas, and stomach.

PLEASE use with caution

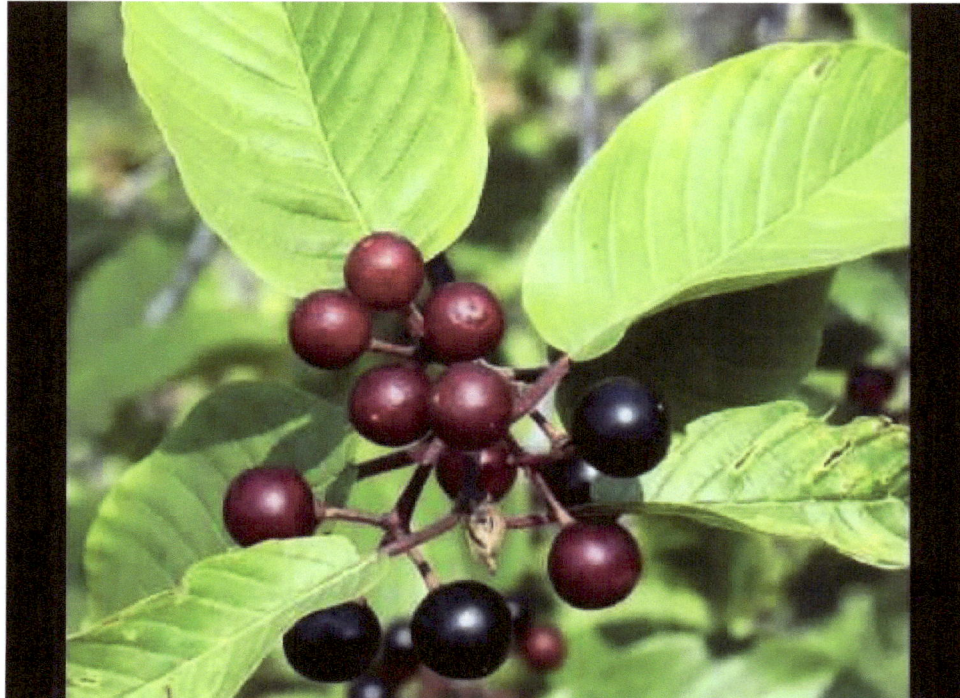

Fennel

Bitter Fennel, Common Fennel

Foeniculum vulgare

Parts Used: Seeds (Tincture, Infusion)

Native to Mediterranean Region

Enhances appetite, digestion and absorption; aids digestion of fatty foods; added to laxative blends to ease griping; stabilizes blood-sugar levels and reduces sugar cravings; settles the stomach; relieves hiccups, colic, bloating, nausea and vomiting, indigestion, heartburn, diarrhea, irritable bowel syndrome, arthritis, gout; diuretic; relieves period pain; regulates the menstrual cycle, amenorrhea, endometriosis, low libido, PMS, menopause.

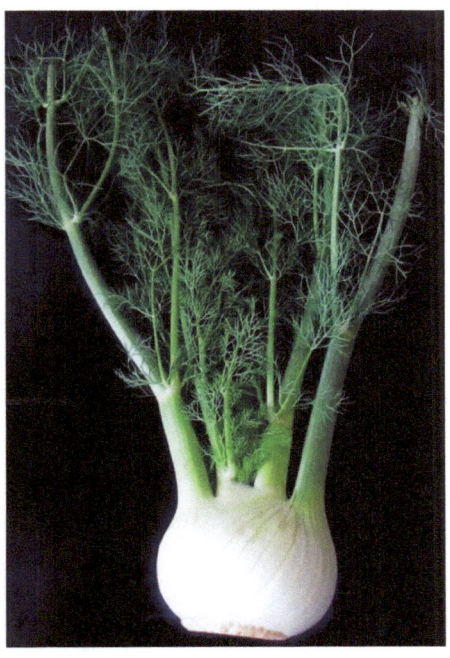

Gentian Root

Wild Gentian, Yellow Gentian, Gentian

Gentiana lutea

Part Used: Root (Tincture)

Native to the high pastures of Central and Southern Europe and Western Asia

Stimulates appetite and digestion, particularly of protein and fats; aids absorption of essential minerals and vitamins; improves the elimination of waste; stimulates bile flow; promotes peristalsis; helpful in poor appetite, nausea, indigestion; anti-inflammatory; cools in gastritis and colitis; clears worms and infections; eases arthritis and gout; antipyretic; induces periods; regulates menstruation; nerve tonic for PMS and menopausal mood swings.

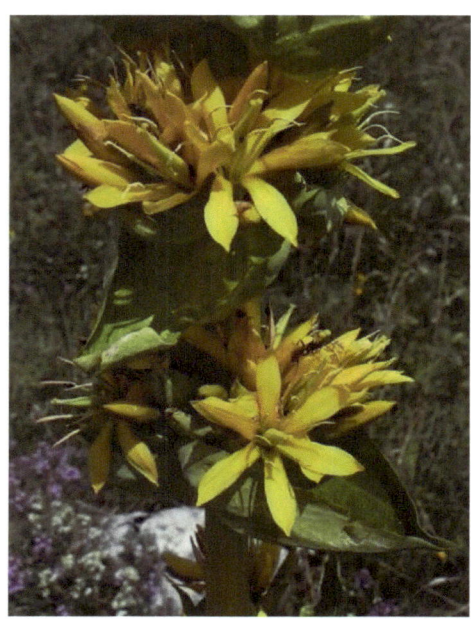

Licorice — Digestive, Respiratory, Reproductive

Gancao, Glycyrrhiza, Sweet Root, Yasti-Madhu

Glycyrrhiza glabra

Parts Used: Pealed Root (Tincture, Decoction), Powdered Root (Infusion)

Native to Europe, Asia, North and South America

Soothes sore throat and dry cough; expectorant; soothes asthma and chest infections; anti-allergenic for hay fever, conjunctivitis, bronchial asthma; lowers stomach acids; relieves heartburn, indigestion, ulcers; mild laxative; increases bile flow from the liver; useful in chronic hepatitis and cirrhosis; improves resistance to physical and mental stress; antiviral for cytomegalovirus and herpes; eases arthritis, eczema, psoriasis. It has estrogenic along with other steroidal properties used to normalize hormone production. It treats adrenal exhaustion and menopausal dysfunction. It is more effective when used with other herbs.

Don't use on anyone with high blood pressure.

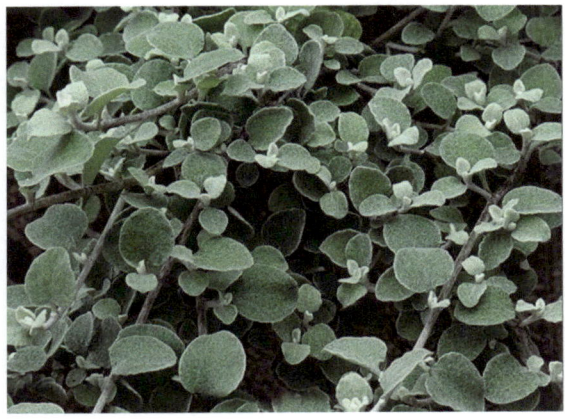

Peppermint

Mantha piperita

Parts Used: Leaf (Tincture, Infusion, Capsules)

Relieves pain and spasms in stomach aches, colic, flatulence, heartburn, indigestion, hiccups, constipation, Irritable Bowel Syndrome and diarrhea; enhances appetite and digestion; relieves nausea, travel sickness; protects stomach lining from irritation and infection, Crohn's disease, Ulcerative colitis; eases tension headaches, joint and muscle pain; clears airways and reduces spasms in asthma; helps against with colds, flu, fevers, H. Pylori, Salmonella Enteritidis, E. Coli, candida, menstrual pain and cramps.

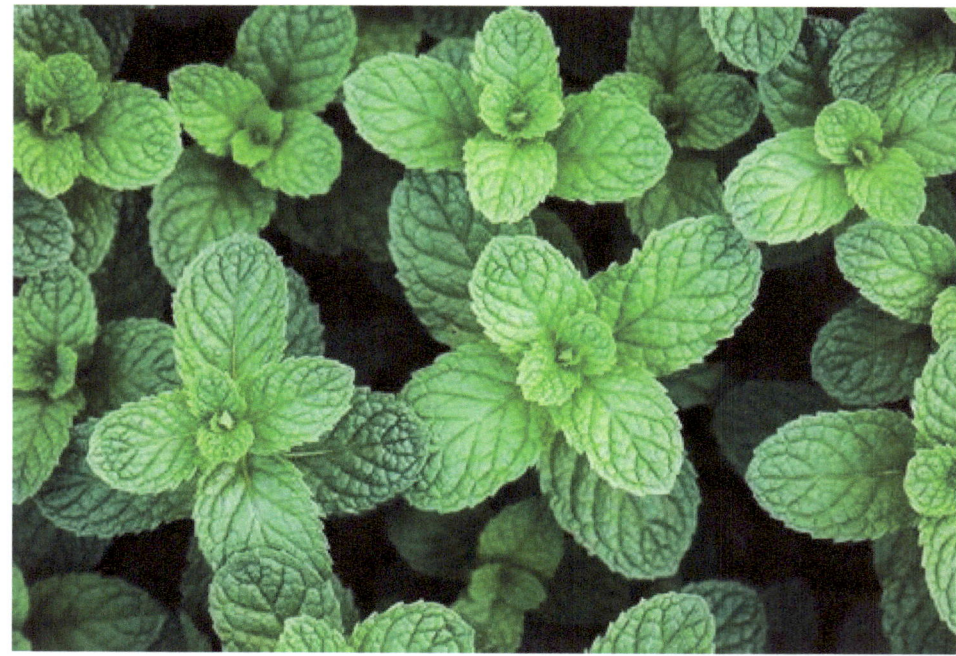

Stinging Nettle   **Alterative, Digestive, Reproductive**

Garden Nettle

Urtica dioica

Parts Used: Leaves, Roots (Infusion-leaf, Tincture-root)

Native to Europe, Asia, North Africa, North America

Protects stomach lining from irritation and infection; relieves diarrhea and flatulence; stimulates liver and kidney function; clears toxins; reduces blood sugar, cough, hay fever, bronchitis, asthma, allergies; stimulates breast milk production; regulates periods and reduces heavy bleeding; rich in Iron; diuretic; prevents incontinence; reduces uric acid for gout; reduces eczema; heals cuts, wounds, hemorrhoids, bites/stings.

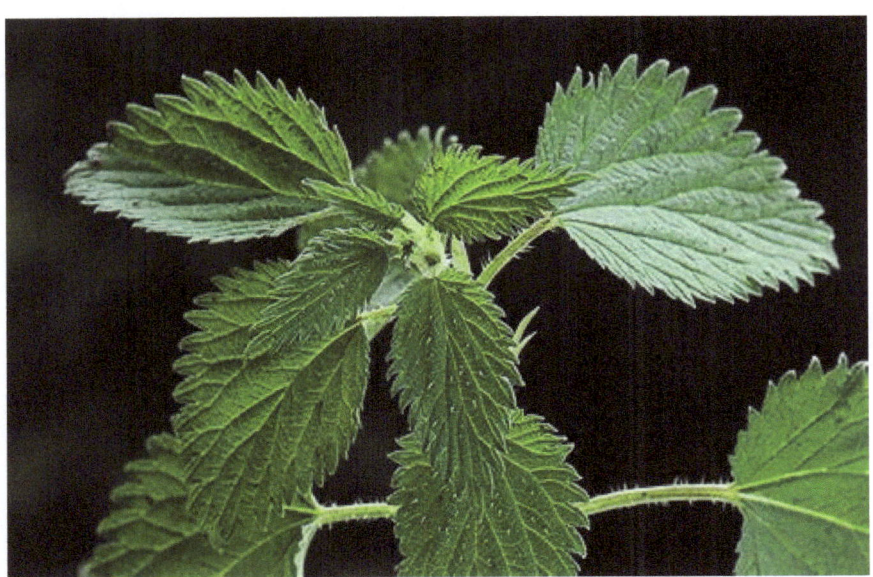

NERVINES

California Poppy

Eschschaizia californica

Parts Used: Ariel Parts (Tincture)

Native to North America

Safe for adults and children as a sedative, helps with anxiety, ADD and ADHD, migraines, sleeping problems in adults and children; anti-spasmodic; helpful in withdrawal from alcohol or tobacco addiction; eases colic.

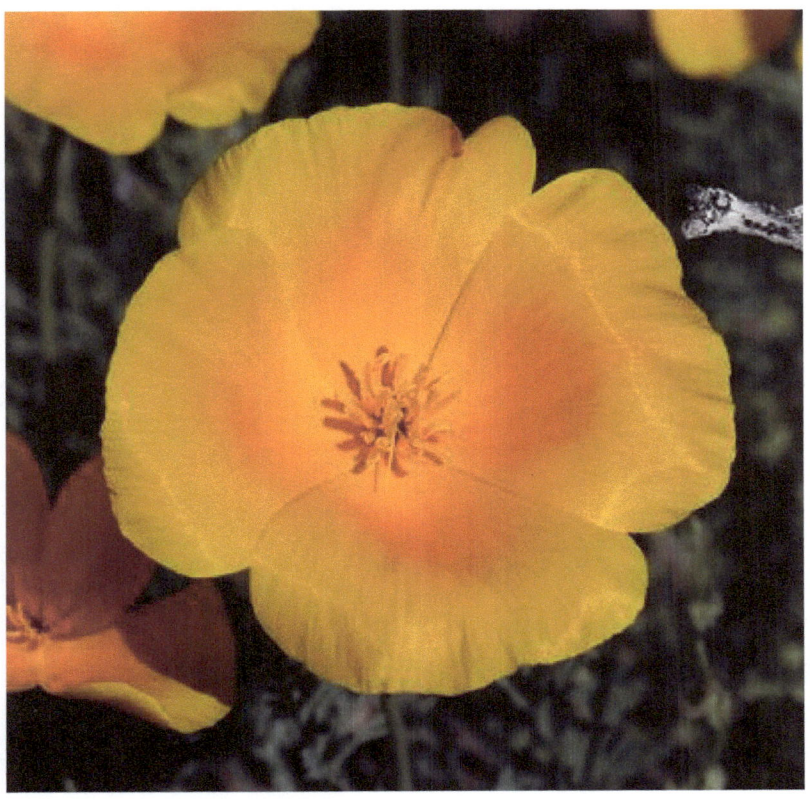

Catnip

Catmint, Nep, Catnep

Nepeta cataria

Parts Used: Leaves and Flowering Tops (Infusion)

Native to Europe, Naturalized in North America

Decreases anxiety, children's colds, diarrhea; diaphoretic; analgesic; fever reducer; promotes sleep, reduces cramps.

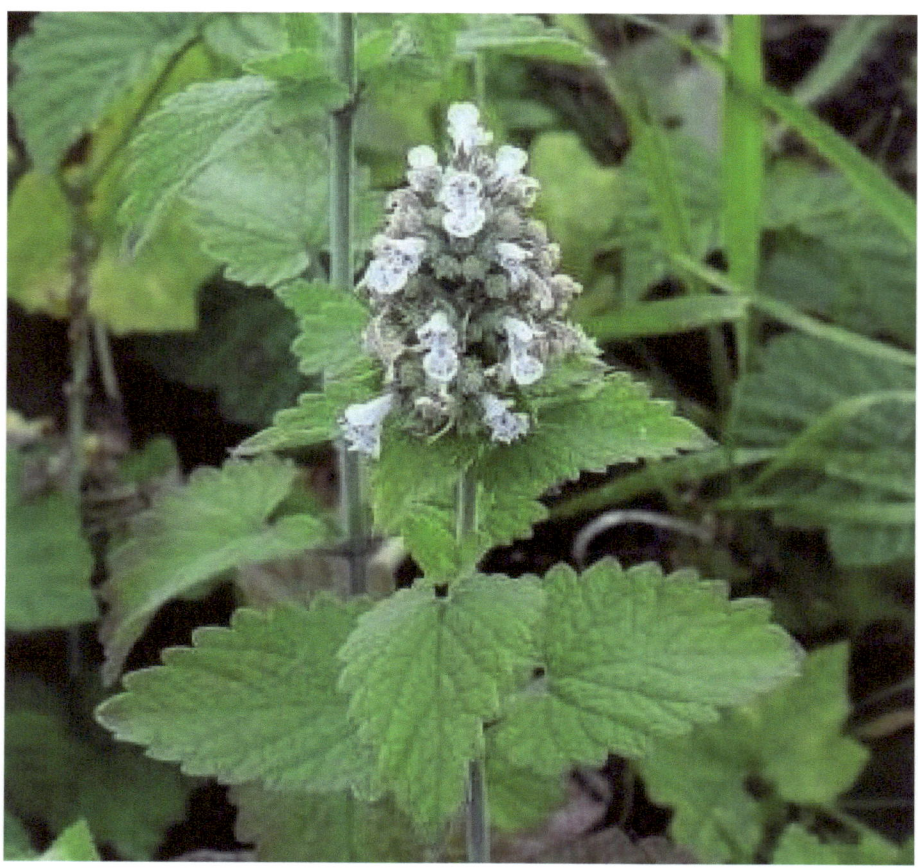

Chamomile

Camomile, Chamomilla, German Chamomila

Chamaemelum nobile (Roman), *Matricaria recutita* (German)

Parts Used- Flower (Tincture, Infusion)

Native to Europe and Northern Asia

Calms anxiety and tension; eases stress; soothes stress-related digestive upsets; enhances immunity; effective remedy for delayed menstruation and irregular menstruation; alleviates premenstrual pain; soothes inflamed/irritable bladder; decreases teething pain, colic; diaphoretic, aids in indigestion, heartburn, acidity; anti-spasmodic; anti-inflammatory.

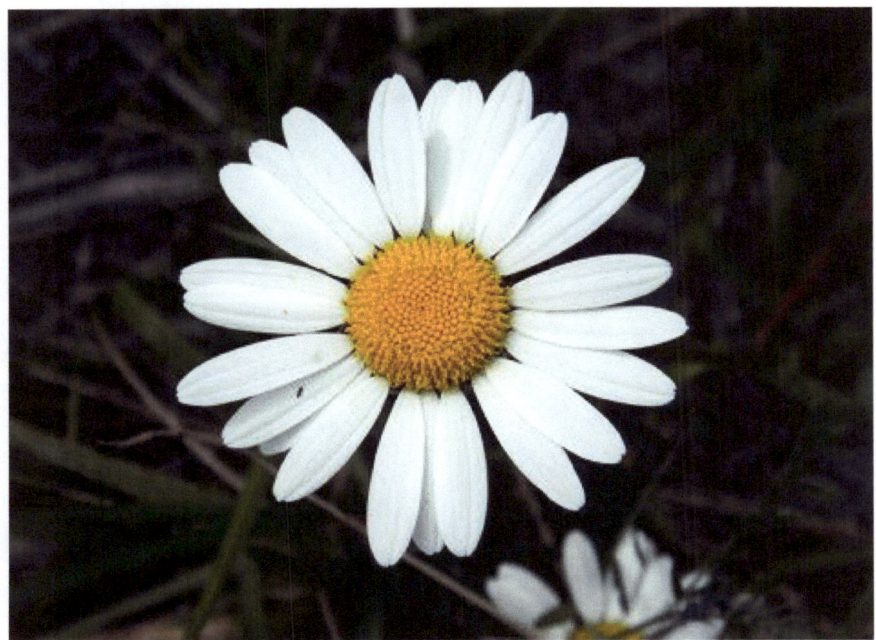

Kava-Kava

Kava, Awa

Parts Used: Root (Decoction)

Native to the Islands of the South Pacific

Aids in reducing nervous anxiety, stress, restlessness; pain reliever; muscle relaxer; anti-depressant; helps with insomnia and headaches.

Do not consume large amounts. It can cause liver damage

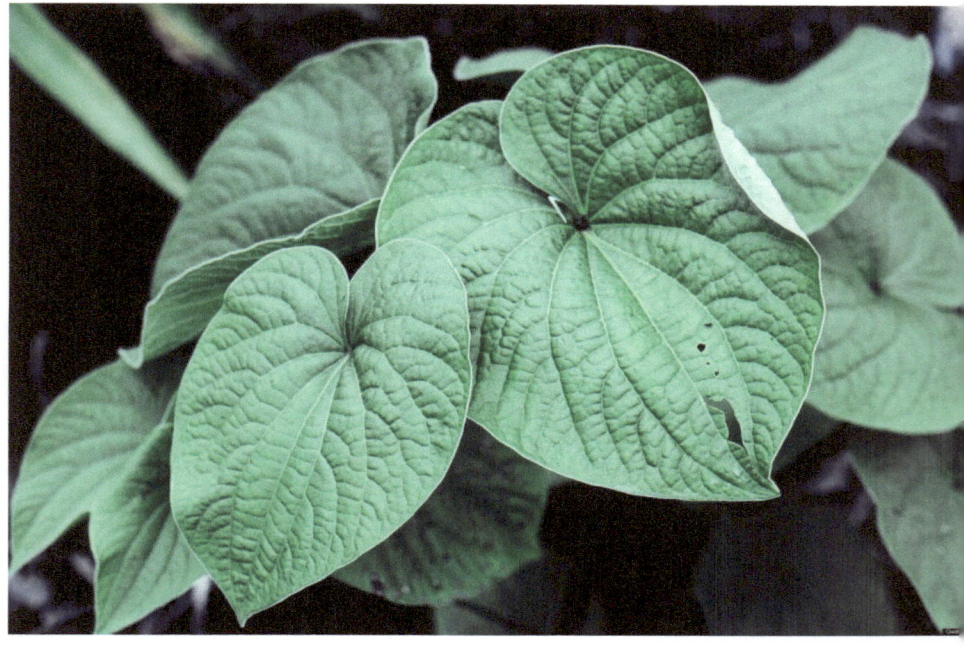

Lavender

English Lavender, Garden Lavender, True Lavender

Lavender officinalis

Parts Used: Flowers (Tincture, Infusion)

Native to Europe

Aids in reducing anxiety, insomnia, Irritable Bowel Syndrome, insect bites, headaches, tension, stress, digestive disturbance; sedative; oil-based for inflamed mosquito bites; essential oil for burns; analgesic.

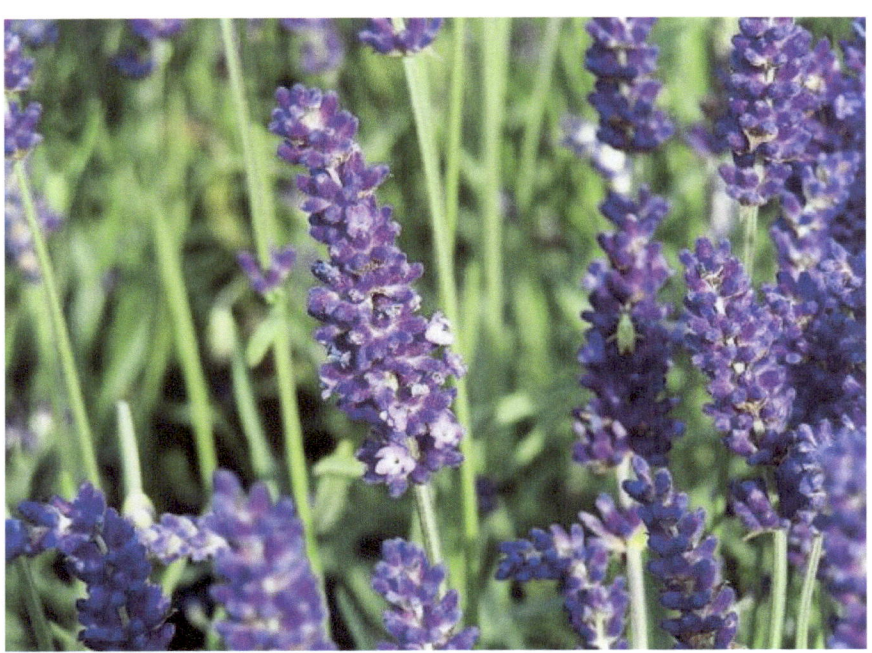

Lemon Balm

Balm, Common Balm, Melissa, Sweet Balm

Melissa officinalis

Parts Used: Leaf (Tincture, Infusion, Capsules)

Native to the Eastern Mediterranean Region and Western Asia, widely cultivated throughout much of Europe

Used of an anti-depressive, anti-spasmodic; reduces nervous sleeping disorder; relieves gas; treats cold sores, anxiety, tension headaches and palpitations; digestive stimulate; topical anti-viral; relieves gas, colic; antihistamine.

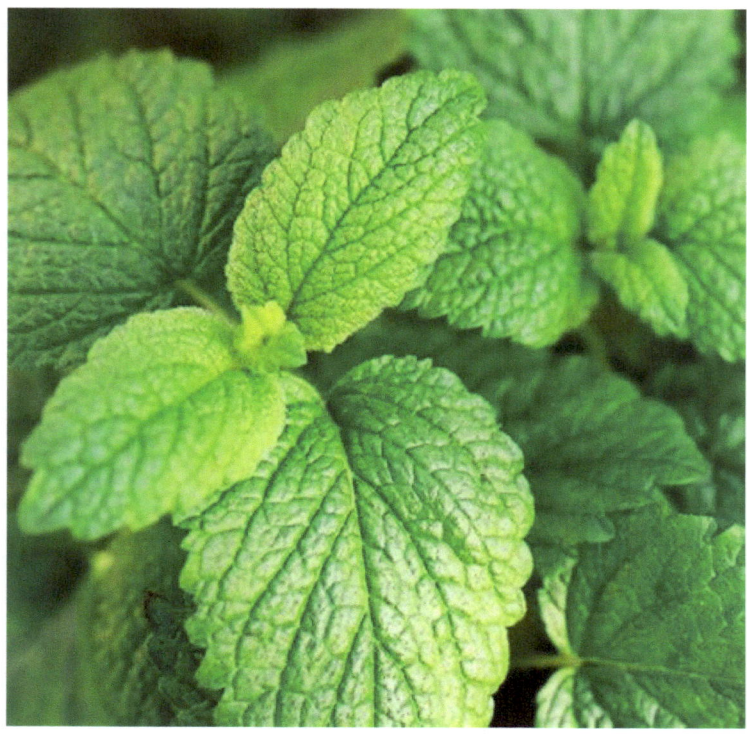

Passion Flower

Maypop Passion Flower, Passifloral, , Passion Vine

Passifloral incarnata

Parts Used: Ariel Parts (Tincture)

Native to the Tropical and Semi Tropical Southeastern United States, Mexico, and Central and South America

It is used for sleep disorders, restlessness, nervous stress, nervous tachycardia, gastrointestinal disorders of nervous origin, neuralgia, muscle twitching, cramps, high blood pressure, colic; mild analgesic; anti-spasmodic.

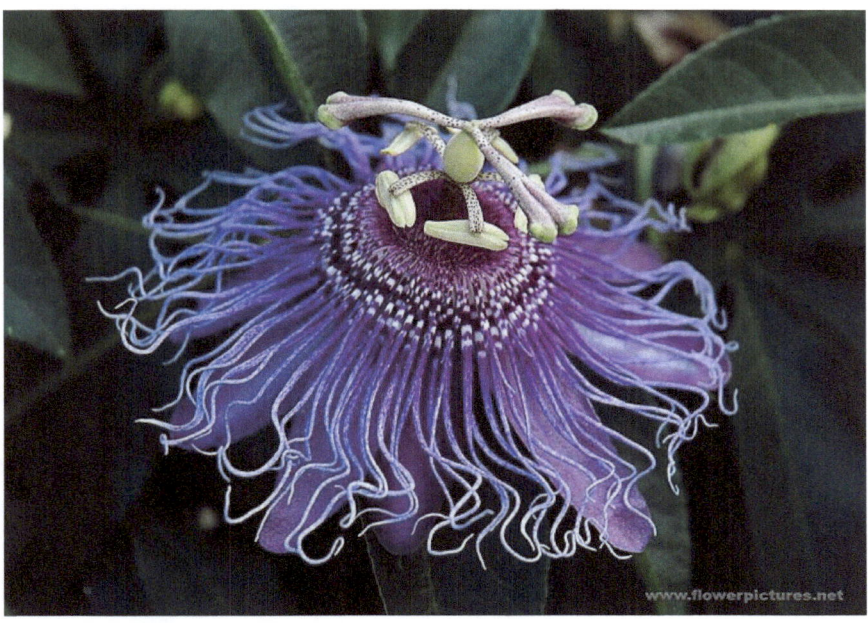

St. John's Wart

Hypericum, Klamath Weed

Hypericum perforatum

Parts Used: Flowering Tops (Tincture, Infusion)

Native to Europe, North Africa, and Western Asia

It grows wild in neglected fields, dry pastures, rangelands, and along country roads.

Used for mild to moderate depression, restlessness, anxiety, irritability, Seasonal Affective Disorder, jetlag, gastritis, sleep disturbance, stomach ulcer, toothache, Sciatica, Shingles, wound healing, arthritis; astringent; analgesic; anti-inflammatory; stimulates liver detoxification; dulls nerve pain; speeds tissue repair.

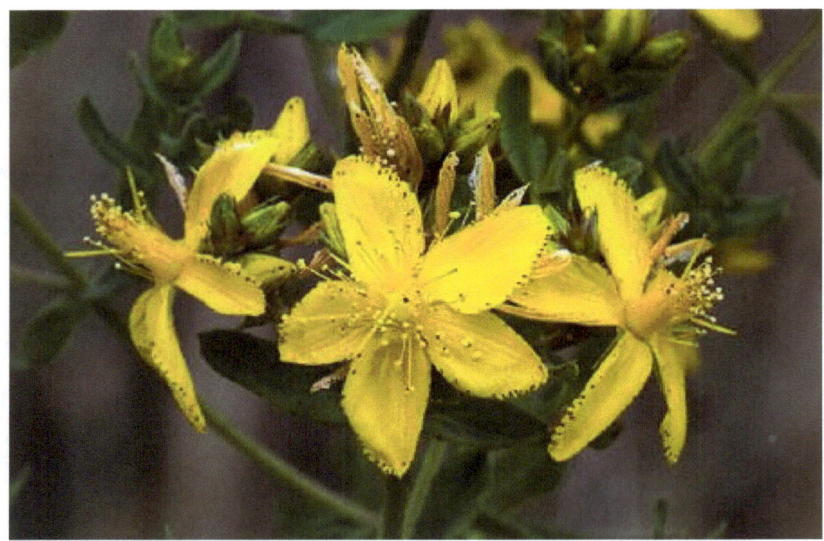

RESPIRATORY

Cayenne

Bell Pepper, Chili Pepper, Red Pepper, Sweet Pepper, Paprika

Capsium annum

Parts Used: Fruit (Tincture, Infusion, Capsules)

Native to Tropical Regions of the Americas

Helps with congestion, infection, inflammation, winter colds, Neuralgia, severe itching, arthritis, rheumatism; clears sinuses.

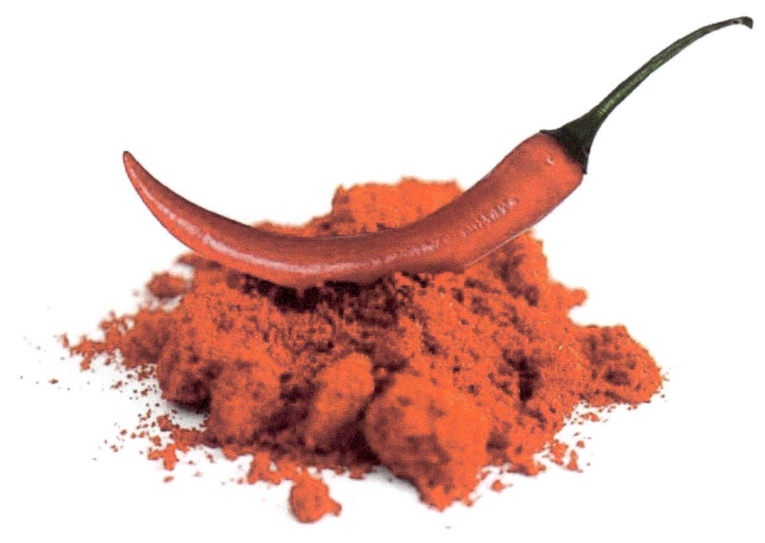

Horehound

White Horehound

Marrubium vulgare

Parts Used: Leaf (Tincture, Infusion)

Native to Europe, Asia, and North Africa

Stimulates appetite and digestion; promotes flow of bile; laxative; eases indigestion, colic, gastroenteritis, diarrhea, intestinal worms; calms palpitations, arterial dilation, anemia; anti-bacterial; anti-spasmodic; expectorant remedy for coughs, colds, flu; relieves croup, asthma, bronchitis, laryngitis, tonsillitis, pneumonia, TB, whooping cough; stimulates the uterus; brings on menstruation in delayed periods and amenorrhea.

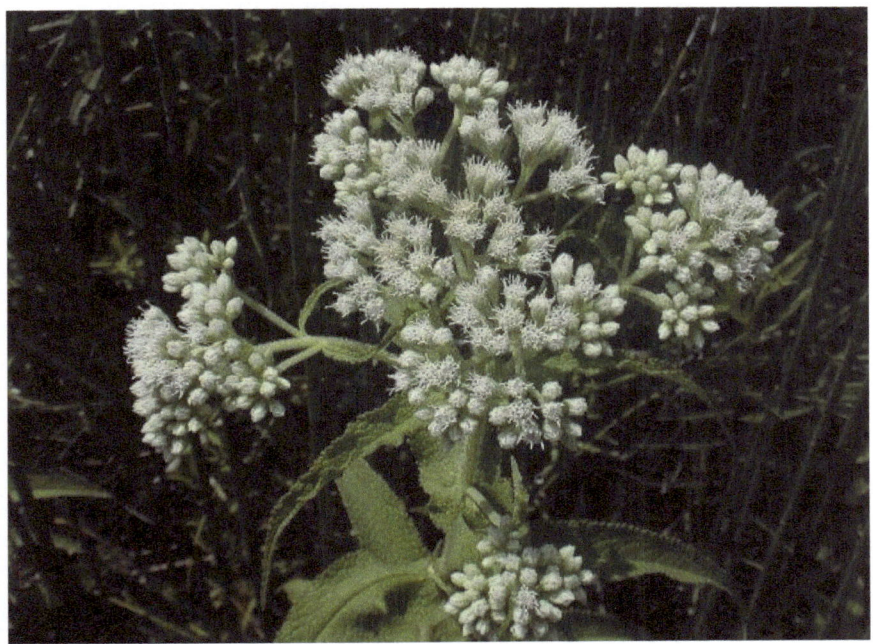

Licorice   Digestive, Respiratory, Reproductive

Gancao, Glycyrrhiza, Sweet Root, Yasti-Madhu

Glycyrrhiza glabra

Parts Used: Pealed Root (Tincture, Decoction), Powdered Root (Infusion)

Native to Europe, Asia, North and South America

Soothes sore throat and dry cough; expectorant; soothes asthma and chest infections; anti-allergenic for hay fever, conjunctivitis, bronchial asthma; lowers stomach acids; relieves heartburn, indigestion, ulcers; mild laxative; increases bile flow from the liver; useful in chronic hepatitis and cirrhosis; improves resistance to physical and mental stress; antiviral for cytomegalovirus and herpes; eases arthritis, eczema, psoriasis. It has estrogenic along with other steroidal properties used to normalize hormone production. It treats adrenal exhaustion and menopausal dysfunction. It is more effective when used with other herbs.

Don't use on anyone with high blood pressure.

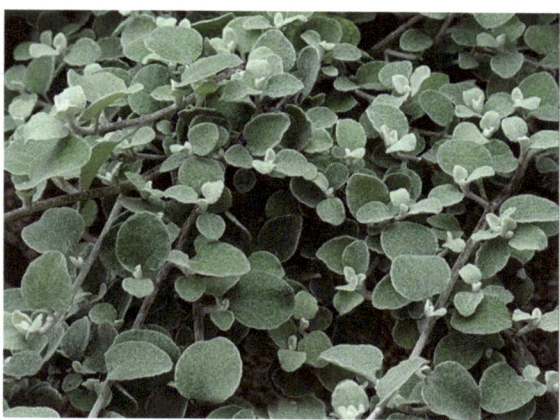

Marshmallow Root

Althaca Root

Althea officinalis

Parts Used: Root, Leaf, Flower (Root-Decoction, Leaf & Flower-Infusion)

Native to Europe, Western Asia

Mild expectorant; immune enhancer; soothes harsh, dry coughs, sore throat, laryngitis, bronchitis and croup, ulcerative colitis, gastritis, peptic ulcers, heartburn, Irritable Bowel Syndrome; reduces peristalsis and relieves diarrhea; stimulates production of white blood cells; relieves cystitis, urethritis and irritable bladder; stimulates flow of breast milk; eases passing of kidney stones.

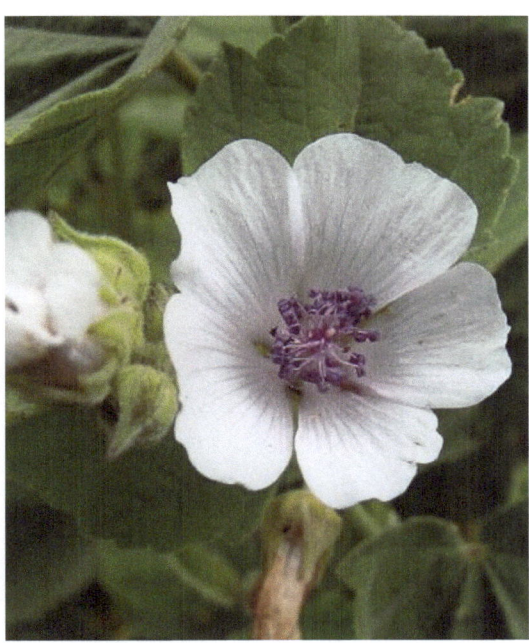

Mullein

Large-Flowered Mullein

Verbascum thapsus

Parts Used: Leaf, Flower, Root (Tincture, Infusion, Capsules)

Native to Europe, Asia, and North Africa

Soothing expectorant for harsh, dry cough, sore throats and inflammatory conditions such as pharyngitis, tracheitis, bronchitis and bronchiectasis; traditional remedy for TB, whooping cough and pleurisy; antiseptic; relieves colds, flu, asthma, croup and chest infections; decongestant; clears phlegm, sinusitis and hay fever; enhances immunity; anti-inflammatory; relieves the pain of swollen glands and mumps; anti-bacterial and anti-viral activity against flu strains and Herpes Simplex; soothing diuretic.

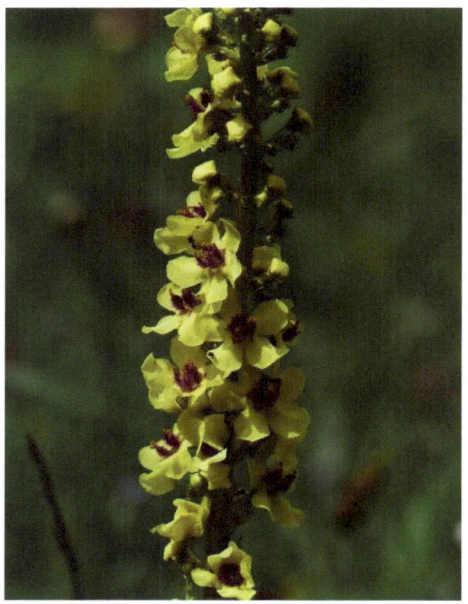

Sage   **Respiratory & Reproductive**

Common Sage, Garden Sage, True Sage

Salvia officinalis

Parts Used: Leaves (Tincture, Infusion)

Native to Southern Europe and the Mediterranean

Decongestant; anti-microbial; expectorant; soothes colds and chest infections; improves appetite, digestion and absorption; relieves bloating and flatulence; beneficial effect on the liver and pancreatic function; lowers blood sugar; reduces anxiety; lifts depression; anti-bacterial; anti-viral for colds, flu, fevers, sore throats, chest infections, Candida, Herpes Simplex 2; elimination of toxins via the kidneys; soothes arthritis and gout; balances hormones; anti-spasmodic for irregular, scanty and painful periods; helps with menopausal night sweats and insomnia; reduces excessive lactation and vaginal discharge; relief of emotional swings, and menstrual flooding.

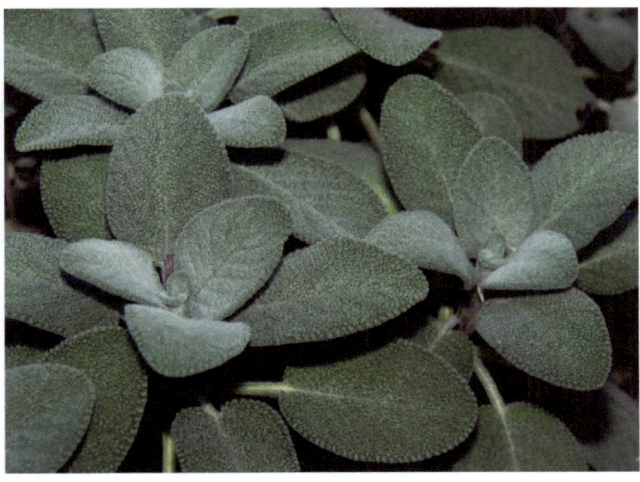

REPRODUCTIVE

American Ginseng

Panax quinquefolius

Parts Used: Root (Decoction, Tincture, Capsules)

Native to Eastern North America and Canada

Stimulates immune system; regulates blood sugar, cholesterol levels, anemia; increases energy, strength and stamina; balances hormones in women during menopause; helps with mood swings, depression, long-term deficiencies and imbalances, fatigue; stress reliever. In men: it helps improve sexual function; increases sexual vitality; treats erectile dysfunction and low sperm count.

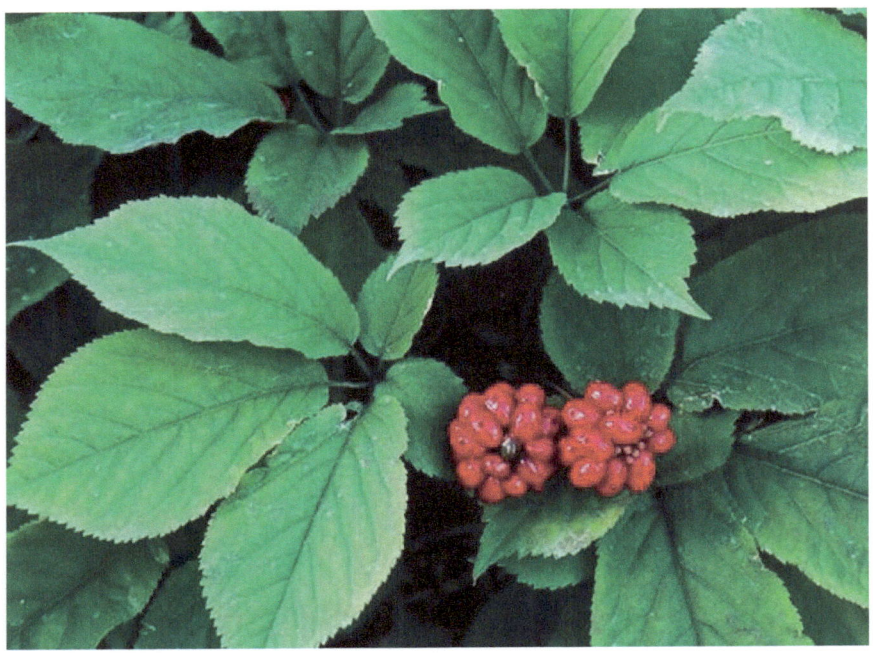

Ashwaganda   *Adaptogen & Reproductive*

Winter Cherry, Indian Ginseng

Parts Used: Root (Capsules, Powder)

Native to India

Helps with stress, anxiety, depression, panic attacks, insomnia, behavioral problems, poor memory, concentration, ADHD, loss of energy and muscular strength, arthritis and insomnia due to advanced age; slows aging process; boosts male virility hindered by age and decreased testosterone levels; anti-inflammatory for joint problems; enhances immunity; promotes sleep.

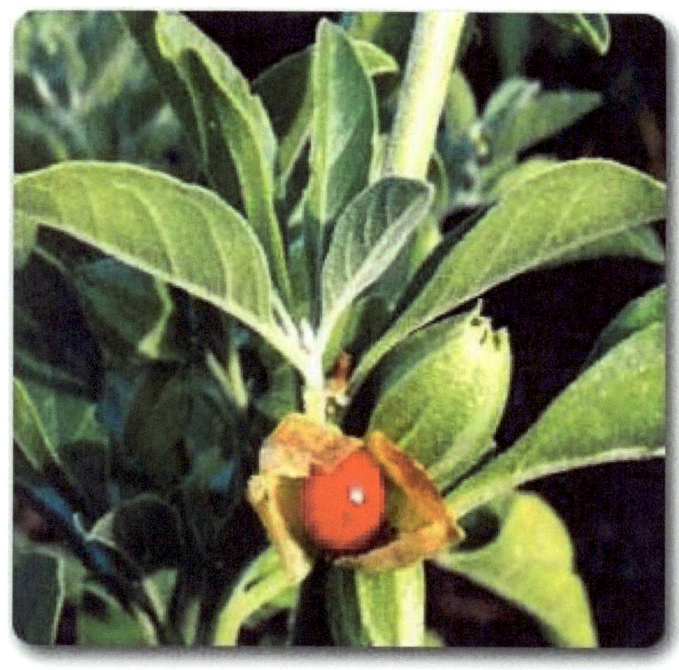

Black Cohosh

Black Snake Root, Bug Wart, Rattle Root, Rattle Weed, Squaw Rootegilate menstrual

Cimicfuga racemosa

Parts Used: Roots, Rhizome (Tincture, Decoction)

Regulates menstrual cycles; relieves PMS, breast pain and swelling, menstrual cramps; relaxes tense uterine muscles, tones uterine muscles when weak; reduces heavy bleeding; eases menopausal symptoms such as anxiety, depression, hot flashes, night sweats, headaches, palpitations, dizziness, vaginal atrophy, low libido.

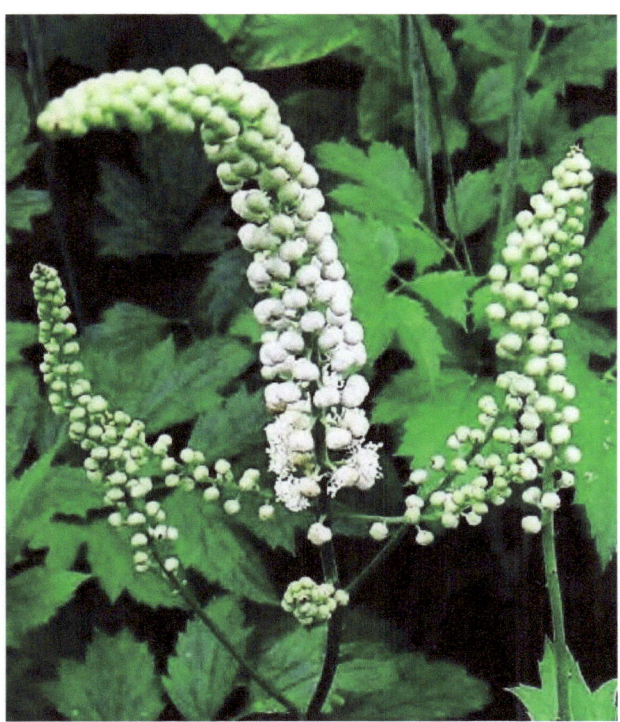

Chaste tree

Chasteberry, monk's pepper

Vitex agnus castus

Parts Used: Fruit (Tincture, Infusion, Capsules)

Native to Mediterranean and Europe

Helps to increase lactation; enhances the natural production of progesterone and luteinizing hormone by stimulating the pituitary gland; diminishes the release of follicle stimulating hormone in order to enhance and allow the normalization of progesterone; helps with infertility, endometriosis, fibroids, womb-lining inflammation, uterine bleeding, impotence, prostatitis, hot flashes, heavy menstrual bleeding; regulates the menstrual cycle.

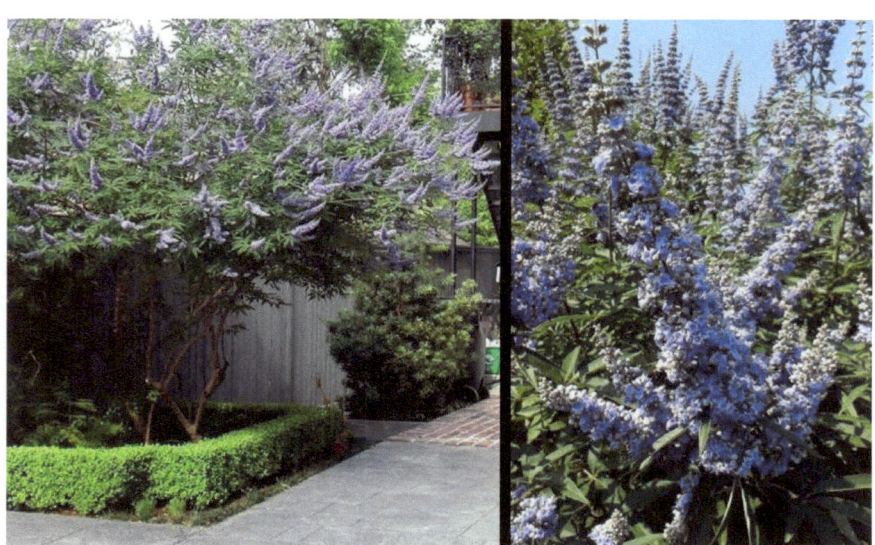

Cramp Bark

Viburnum opulus

Parts Used: Bark (Tincture, Decoction)

Native to Europe, North America, and Northern Asia

Relaxes uterine muscles in overly strong contractions; eases menstrual cramping and pain; prevents excessive menstrual blood flow.

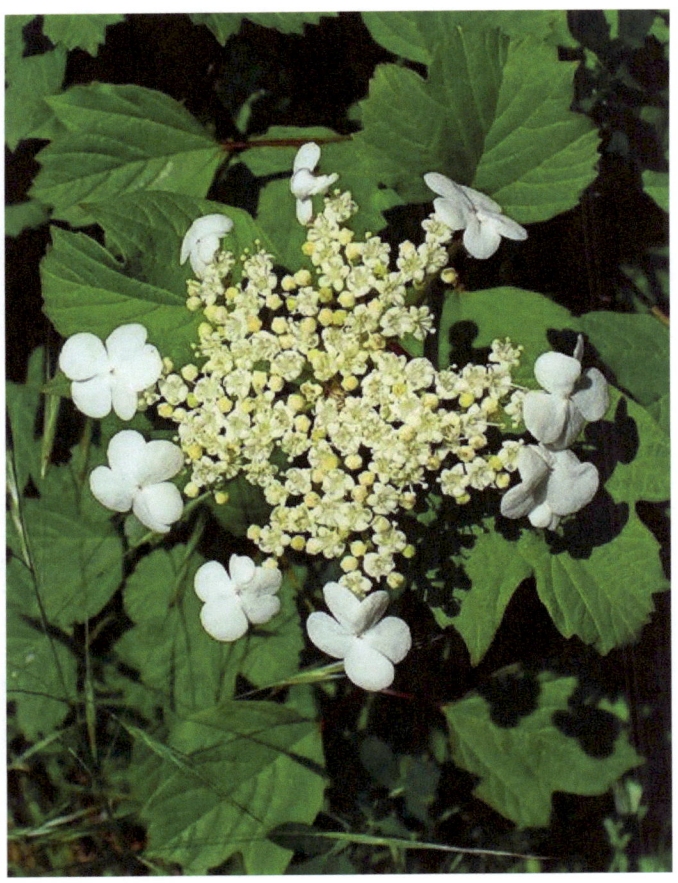

Dong Quai

Chinese Angelica, Dang Gui, Toki, Women's Ginseng

Angelica sinensis

Parts Used: Roots (Tincture, Capsules)

Native to Japan, China, and Korea

Tones the reproductive organs and helps to make an easier hormonal transition during menopause by acting as a hormonal regulator; relieves hot flashes; alleviates vaginal dryness, insomnia and palpitations related to menopause.

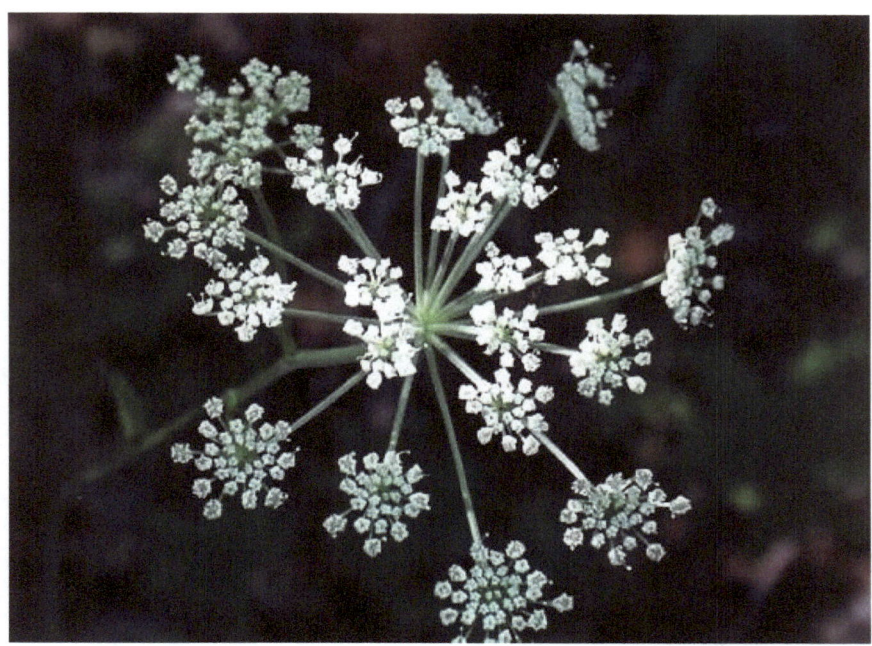

Fenugreek
Bird's Foot, Greek Hayseed, Trigonella

Trigonella foenum-graecum

Parts Used: Seeds (Tincture, Decoction, Capsules)

Native to Europe And Asia

Reduces menopausal symptoms, hot flashes, night sweats, vaginal dryness, depression and insomnia; stimulates milk flow in nursing mothers; an aphrodisiac; promotes fertility.

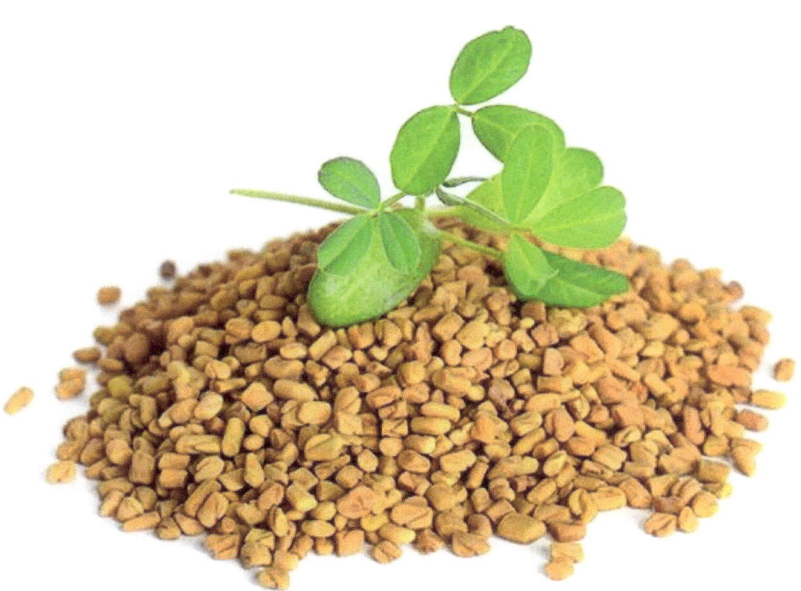

Licorice   **Digestive, Respiratory, Reproductive**

Gancao, Glycyrrhiza, Sweet Root, Yasti-Madhu

Glycyrrhiza glabra

Parts Used: Pealed Root (Tincture, Decoction), Powdered Root (Infusion)

Native to Europe, Asia, North and South America

Soothes sore throat and dry cough; expectorant; soothes asthma and chest infections; anti-allergenic for hay fever, conjunctivitis, bronchial asthma; lowers stomach acids; relieves heartburn, indigestion, ulcers; mild laxative; increases bile flow from the liver; useful in chronic hepatitis and cirrhosis; improves resistance to physical and mental stress; antiviral for cytomegalovirus and herpes; eases arthritis, eczema, psoriasis. It has estrogenic along with other steroidal properties used to normalize hormone production. It treats adrenal exhaustion and menopausal dysfunction. It is more effective when used with other herbs.

Don't use on anyone with high blood pressure.

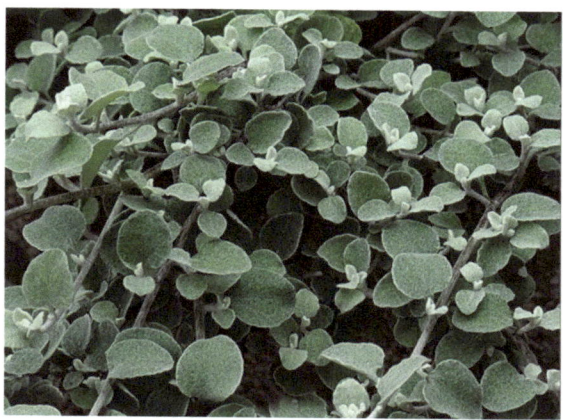

Mother Wart

Lion's Tail, Lion's Tart, Throw Wart

Leonurus cardiaca

Parts Used: Flower Tops, Leaves (Tincture, Infusion, Capsules)

Native to Europe, Canada, and the United States

Regulates rapid heart rate; strengthens the heart muscle; used for arteriosclerosis; dissolves blood clots; lowers blood pressure; anti-depressive; lessens severity of hot flashes; relieves insomnia; reduces menstrual cramps, menopausal palpitations, uterine pain; restores thickness and the elasticity of the vaginal wall; enhances fertility; increases libido; prevents post-partum infection; helps prevent postpartum depression; stimulates menstruation; helps with menstrual headaches.

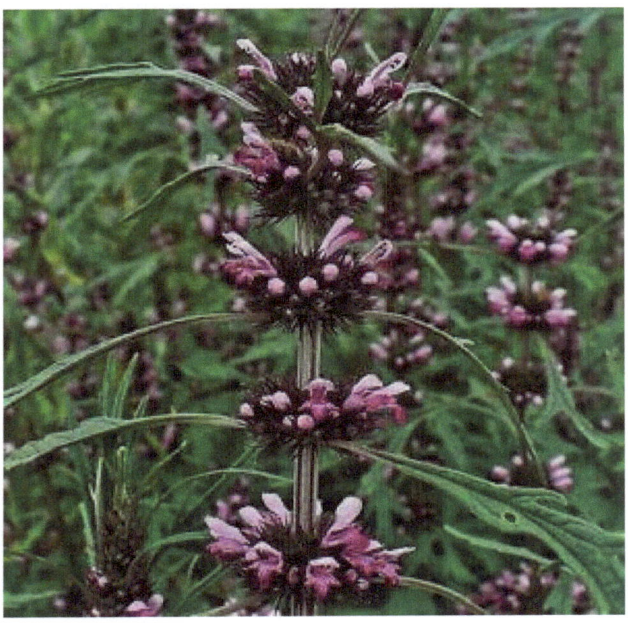

Red Clover Blossoms

Trifollium pretense

Parts Used- Flower (Tincture, Infusion, Capsule)

Native to United States, Europe

Helps with hot flashes, night sweats, headaches, poor sleep; heart-healthy application during and after menopause.

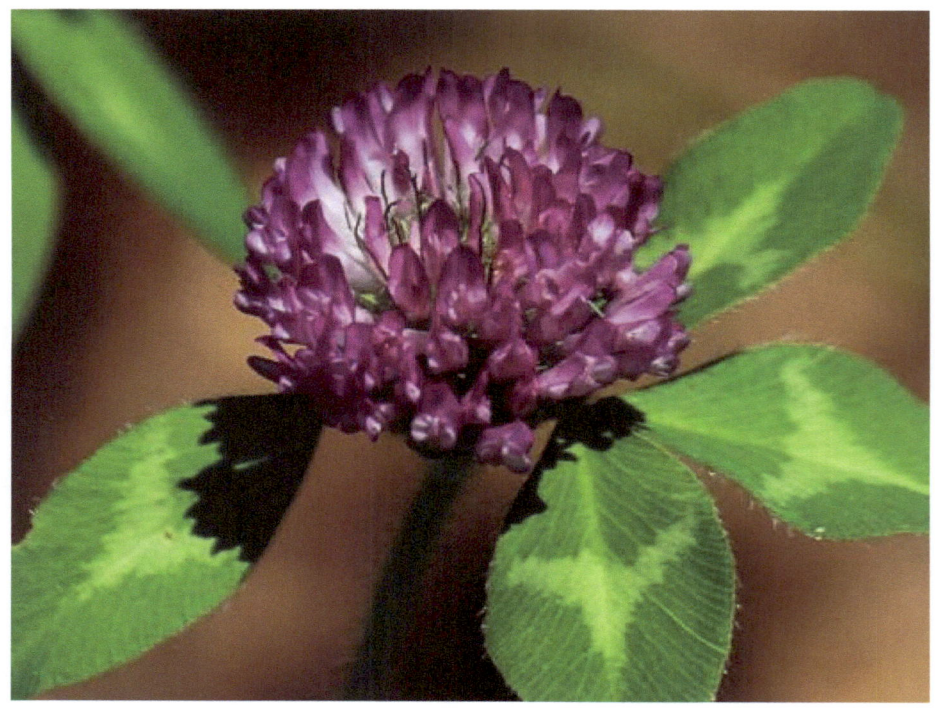

Red Raspberry Leaf
Bramble, Red Raspberry

Rubus idaeus

Parts Used: Leaves (Infusion, Tincture, Capsules)

Native to Europe, North America, and Asia

It provides Iron, Vitamin C, Potassium, Vitamin B and E, Calcium which are beneficial to a woman during pregnancy; decreases uterine swelling; reduces postpartum bleeding; prevents miscarriage; increases milk flow after birth; reduces morning sickness; speeds the labor process.

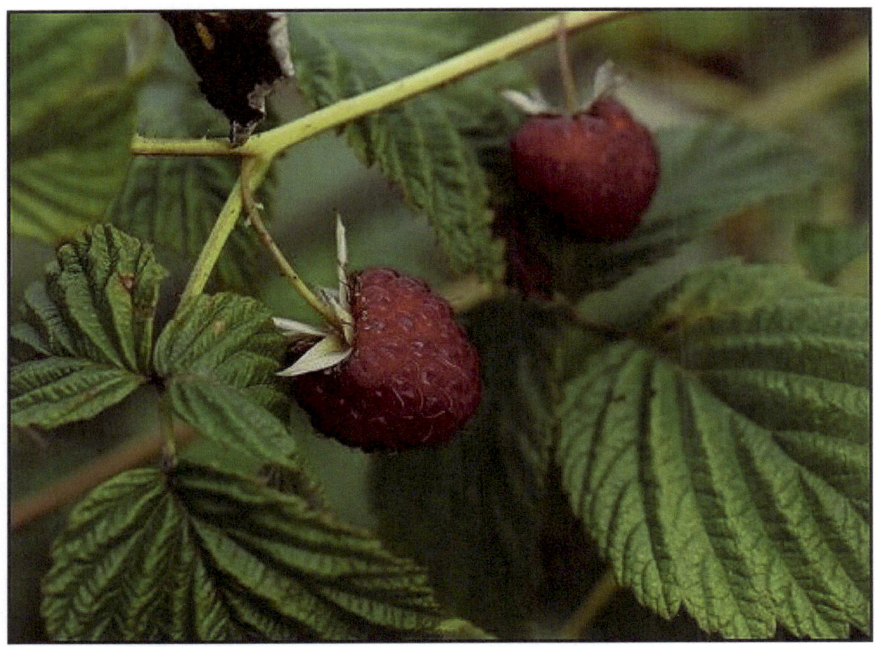

Sage   **Respiratory & Reproductive**

Common Sage, Garden Sage, True Sage

Salvia officinalis

Parts Used: Leaves (Tincture, Infusion)

Native to Southern Europe and the Mediterranean

Decongestant; anti-microbial; expectorant; soothes colds and chest infections; improves appetite, digestion and absorption; relieves bloating and flatulence; beneficial effect on the liver and pancreatic function; lowers blood sugar; reduces anxiety; lifts depression; anti-bacterial; anti-viral for colds, flu, fevers, sore throats, chest infections, Candida, Herpes Simplex 2; elimination of toxins via the kidneys; soothes arthritis and gout; balances hormones; anti-spasmodic for irregular, scanty and painful periods; helps with menopausal night sweats and insomnia; reduces excessive lactation and vaginal discharge; relief of emotional swings, and menstrual flooding.

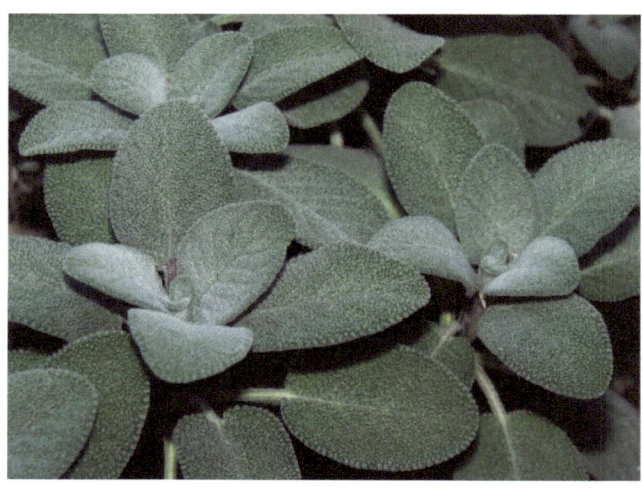

Stinging Nettle   **Alterative, Digestive, Reproductive**

Garden Nettle

Urtica dioica

Parts Used: Leaves, Roots (Infusion-leaf, Tincture-root)

Native to Europe, Asia, North Africa, North America

Protects stomach lining from irritation and infection; relieves diarrhea and flatulence; stimulates liver and kidney function; clears toxins; reduces blood sugar, cough, hay fever, bronchitis, asthma, allergies; stimulates breast milk production; regulates periods and reduces heavy bleeding; rich in Iron; diuretic; prevents incontinence; reduces uric acid for gout; reduces eczema; heals cuts, wounds, hemorrhoids, bites/stings.

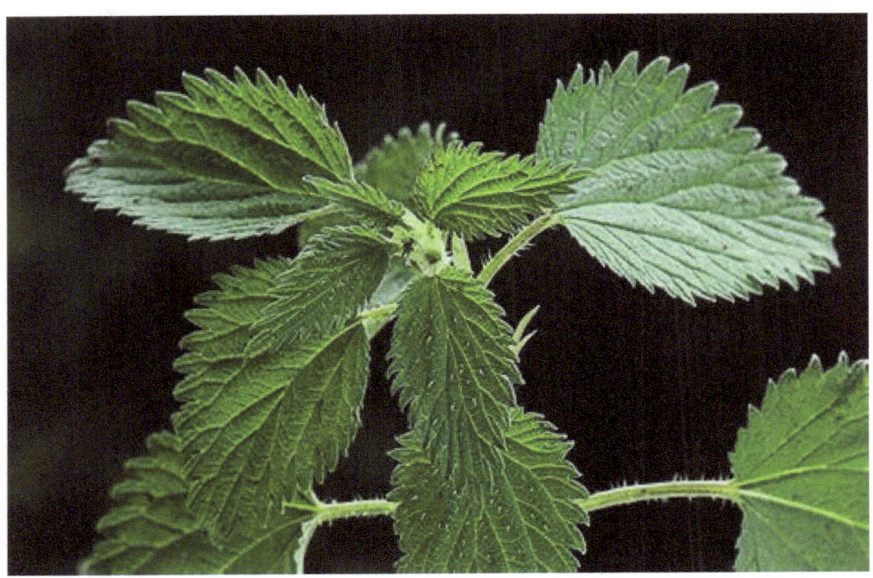

Wild Yam Root

Colic Root, Rheumatism Root, China Root

Dioscorea villosa

Parts Used: Root (Tincture, Decoction, Capsules)

Native to United States and Central America

Acts as a hormone regulator by balancing the ratio of estrogen to progesterone levels in the reproductive system; relieves tension and cramps in the uterus and ovaries; helps with spasmodic dysmenorrhea associated with nausea and ovarian pain.

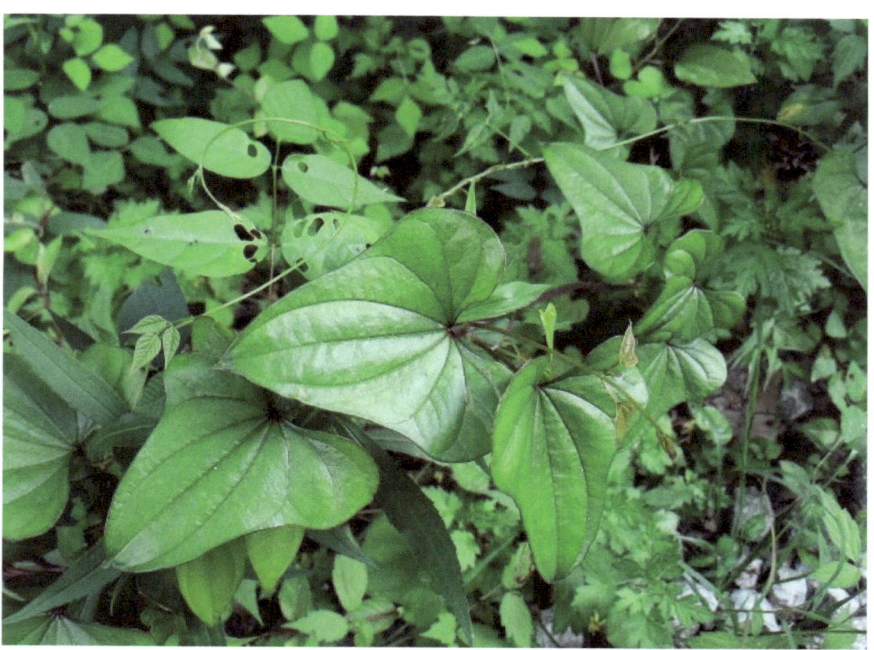

Yarrow

Blood wart, nose bleed

Achillea millefolium

Parts Used: Ariel Parts (Tincture, Infusion, Capsules).

Native to Asia, Europe, and North America

Used to control heavy menstrual bleeding. When the tea is drunk cold or as a tincture, it helps with night sweats and hot flashes.

Do not drink uninterrupted for more than 2 weeks due to the dangers of hepatic inflammation ensuing.

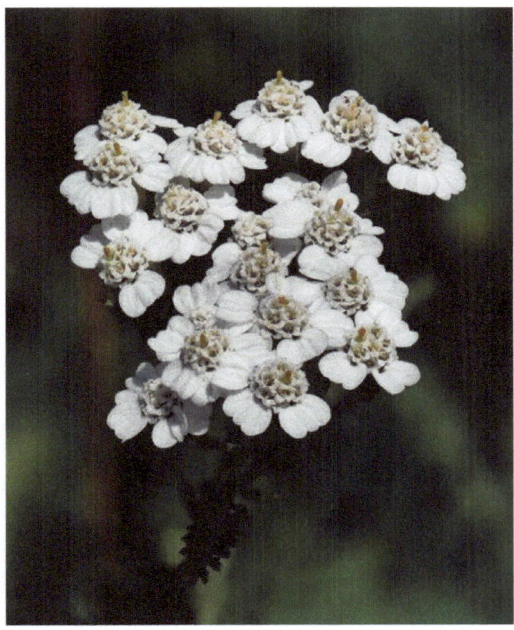

General Index

American Ginseng, 51
Anise Seed, 27
Ashwaganda, 11, 52
Astragalus, 12
Black Cohosh, 53
Burdock Root, 19
California Poppy, 35
Cascara Sagrada, 28
Catnip, 36
Cayenne, 44
Chamomile, 37
Chaste Tree, 54
Cleavers, 13
Cramp Bark, 55
Dandelion, 20
Dong Quai, 56
Echinacea, 21
Eleuthero, 14
Fennel, 29
Fenugreek, 57
Garlic, 22
Gentian Root, 30
Golden Seal, 23
Harvesting, Drying, and Storing Medicinal Herbs, 5
He Shou Wu, 15
Herbal Tincture, 7-8
Herbal Terminology, 1-3
Holy Basil, 16
Horehound, 45
Kava-Kava, 38
Lavender, 39
Lemon Balm, 40
Licorice, 31, 46, 58
Marshmallow Root, 47
Preparing Medicinal Teas, 6

Mother Wart, 59
Mullein, 48
Passion Flower, 41
Peppermint, 32
Red Raspberry Leaf, 61
Red Clover Blossoms, 60
References, 68
Rhodiola, 17
Sage, 49, 62
Salve Making, 9
St. John's Wart, 42
Stinging Nettle, 24, 33, 63
Wild Yam Root, 64
Yarrow, 65
Yellow Dock, 25

References

Alfs, Matthew. (2003). 300 Herbs: Their Indications & Contraindications. Old Theology Book House.

Mcintyre, Anne. (2015). *Herbal Remedies for Everyday Living*. Octopus Publishing Group.

Chevallier, Andrew. (2001). *Herbal Remedies Handbook*. Dorling Kindersley Pub.

Gladstar, Rosemary. (2012) *Medicinal Herbs A Beginner's Guide*. Massachusetts: Storey Publishing.

Wardwell, Joyce A. (1998). *The Herbal Home Remedy Book*. Massachusetts: Storey Publishing.

Zimmermann, Ellen. EZ Herbs.

www.ingramcontent.com/pod-product-compliance
Lightning Source LLC
Chambersburg PA
CBHW040321220526
45473CB00009B/2518